QUEERING FAT EMBODIMENT

Queer Interventions

Series editor:
Michael O'Rourke
Independent Colleges, Dublin

Queer Interventions is an exciting, fresh and unique new series designed to publish innovative, experimental and theoretically engaged work in the burgeoning field of queer studies.

The aim of the series is to interrogate, develop and challenge queer theory, publishing queer work which intersects with other theoretical schools and is accessible whilst valuing difficulty; empirical work which is metatheoretical in focus; ethical and political projects and most importantly work which is self-reflexive about methodological and geographical location.

The series is interdisciplinary in focus and publishes monographs and collections of essays by new and established scholars. The editors intend the series to promote and maintain high scholarly standards of research and to be attentive to queer theory's shortcomings, silences, hegemonies and exclusions. They aim to encourage independence, creativity and experimentation: to make a queer theory that matters and to recreate it as something important; a space where new and exciting things can happen.

Titles in this series:

Queer Futures
Reconsidering Ethics, Activism, and the Political
Edited by Elahe Haschemi Yekani,
Eveline Kilian and Beatrice Michaelis
ISBN: 978-1-4094-3710-9

Hegemony and Heteronormativity
Revisiting 'The Political' in Queer Politics
Edited by María do Mar Castro Varela,
Nikita Dhawan and Antke Engel
ISBN: 978-1-4094-0320-3

Queer in Europe
Contemporary Case Studies
Edited by Lisa Downing and Robert Gillett
ISBN: 978-1-4094-0464-4

Queering Fat Embodiment

Edited by

CAT PAUSÉ
Massey University, New Zealand

JACKIE WYKES
University of Melbourne, Australia

SAMANTHA MURRAY

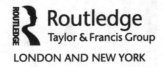

Routledge
Taylor & Francis Group

LONDON AND NEW YORK

First published 2014 by Ashgate Publishing

2 Park Square, Milton Park, Abingdon, Oxfordshire OX14 4RN
52 Vanderbilt Avenue, New York, NY 10017

Routledge is an imprint of the Taylor & Francis Group, an informa business

First issued in paperback 2020

British Library Cataloguing in Publication Data
A catalogue record for this book is available from the British Library

The Library of Congress has cataloged the printed edition as follows:
Queering fat embodiment / [edited] by Cat Pausé, Jackie Wykes and Samantha Murray.
   pages cm. -- (Queer interventions)
 Includes bibliographical references and index.
 ISBN 978-1-4094-6542-3 (hardback)
1. Queer theory. 2. Obesity--Social aspects. 3. Human body--Social aspects. 4.
Identity (Psychology) I. Pausé, Cat. II. Wykes, Jackie. III. Murray, Samantha, 1978-
 HQ76.25.Q3856 2014
 306.7601--dc23

2014000815

ISBN 978-1-4094-6542-3 (hbk)
ISBN 978-0-367-60077-8 (pbk)

Contents

List of Figures

About the Editors

Dr Cat Pausé is a human development lecturer and fat studies researcher at Massey University. Her research focuses on the effects of spoiled identities on the health and well-being of marginalised populations, specifically fat people. Her current projects include an auto-ethnographic exploration of coming out as fat and exploring whether fat people are allowed to have health. Her work has been published in *Human Development* (2007), *Higher Education Research and Development* (2011), *Somatechnics* (2012), and *Feminist Review* (2012). Cat also maintains a presence in the fat-o-sphere with her blog, Tumblr, and podcast, 'Friend of Marilyn'.

Jackie Wykes is a PhD candidate in the School of Culture and Communications at the University of Melbourne, where she also teaches in cultural studies. Her thesis looks at fat embodiment and sexual subjectivity. Her academic work has been published in *Somatechnics* (2012) and she is the co-editor of the forthcoming *Fat Mook* (Vignette Press 2014). She is involved in a range of fat activist projects, including the Melbourne chapter of Aquaporko fat synchronised swim team, Chub Republic, and Va Va Boombah fat burlesque.

Dr Samantha Murray is the author of *The 'Fat' Female Body* (Palgrave Macmillan 2008), and co-editor (with Nikki Sullivan) of *Somatechnics: Queering the Technologisation of Bodies* (Ashgate 2009). Sam has also published numerous articles on fat embodiment, weight loss surgeries, and discourses of normalcy and pathology.

Notes on Contributors

Media networks, censorship, and social control via the body are fundamental research interests for **Dr Scott Beattie**, who is a senior lecturer at Deakin University. Previously, he has examined the way in which internet censorship produces spaces of conformity by idealising a family-friendly model of public space. Scott is also a visual artist who enjoys exploring the contours of all types of bodies and you can find his art blog at sotadic.blogspot.com.

James Burford is a doctoral student at Auckland University, in the School of Critical Studies in Education. He has previously worked as an educator, and as a youth worker and community development practitioner with queer and trans* communities. His research interests stretch from queering international development practice to queer/trans* interventions in secondary and higher education. His doctoral study examines the affective practices of doctoral writers in Aotearoa New Zealand.

Kimberly Dark teaches in the sociology department at California State University, San Marcos. Her public scholarship combines storytelling – both on stage and in print – with cultural critique. *The Advocate* newsmagazine recently named her as one of the top six speakers and performers working with LGBT issues on American university campuses today. She travels internationally, inspiring audiences to become more conscious cultural creators. Learn more about her work, or book a presentation at www.kimberlydark.com.

Zoë Meleo-Erwin received her PhD in sociology from the City University of New York Graduate Center. She holds a previous MA in disability studies from the Graduate Center. Her dissertation research focused on the biosociality of weight loss surgery support groups. Her previous publications appear in *Critical Perspectives on Addiction* (*Advances in Medical Sociology*, 14, 2012), *Feminism and Psychology* (2012), *Health: An Interdisciplinary Journal for the Social Study of Health, Illness and Medicine* (2011), and *International Review of Qualitative Research* (2010). She can be found at www.zoemeleoerwin.com.

Stefanie A. Jones is a PhD student in the theatre program at the CUNY Graduate Center, a Ronald E. McNair scholar, and a writer, educator and critic.

SAJ's areas of interest are sociology of culture, critical race theory, and popular culture in the age of neoliberalism.

Margitte Leah Kristjansson is a PhD student in the Department of Communication at the University of California, San Diego, where her work is focused primarily on fat fashion, fat consumption practices, and examining the queerness of fat embodiment. Her other research interests include fat activism, histories of body regulation, articulating fat culture, and uncovering anti-fat biases in media representations of the fat body. She is also a fat activist, blogger and filmmaker.

Kathleen LeBesco is Associate Dean for Academic Affairs at Marymount Manhattan College. She is the author of *Revolting Bodies? The Struggle to Redefine Fat Identity*, co-author of *Culinary Capital*, and co-editor of *Bodies Out of Bounds? Fatness and Transgression, Edible Ideologies: Representing Food and Meaning, The Drag King Anthology*, and special issues of *The Review of Education, Pedagogy and Cultural Studies* on the teacher's body and *Women and Performance: A Journal of Feminist Theory* on excess. Her work concerns food and popular culture, fat activism, disability and representation, working class identity and queer politics.

Dr Jennifer Lee is a lecturer in creative writing, literary studies and gender studies at Victoria University in Melbourne, Australia. She publishes academic writing, feature articles, fiction and memoir that stem from the intersection of fat studies and creative writing. She is co-editing *Fat Mook* (part magazine, part book) with Jackie Wykes. Jennifer has a long history of curating queer events for Midsumma, the queer arts and culture festival in Melbourne. Her last sold-out event for Midsumma was 'Dangerous Curves Ahead' – eight performers exploring the intersections of fat and queer.

Robyn Longhurst is Professor of Geography at University of Waikato. She has served terms as Editor-in-Chief of *Gender, Place and Culture: A Journal of Feminist Geography* and Chair of the International Geographical Union Commission on Gender and Geography. She teaches feminist, social, and cultural geography. Robyn has published on issues relating to pregnancy, sexuality, mothering, 'visceral geographies', masculinities, and body size and shape. She is author of *Bodies: Exploring Fluid Boundaries* (2001), *Maternities: Gender, Bodies and Spaces* (2008), and co-author of *Pleasure Zones: Bodies, Cities, Spaces* (2001) and *Space, Place, and Sex: Geographies of Sexualities* (2010).

Samuel Orchard is an artist, activist, and queer trans-man. He creates stories about and for queer and trans people that move beyond the common narratives that are propagated by mainstream commercial meanings. He has an LLB/

BA (First Class Hons) in Film, Media and Communication, and an MA (First Class Hons) in Creative Writing. Sam is passionate about youth development programmes and works in the mental health sector.

Acknowledgements

We would like to thank all of the individuals who contributed to this collection, and Ashgate for their commitment in publishing critical scholarship. We especially appreciate the series editor, Michael O'Rourke, who was enthusiastic about the idea from the beginning, and our editor, Neil Jordan, for his guidance and support through the process.

From Sam:

I am thankful for my co-editors, who drove this project and pushed its conceptual boundaries in exciting, unexpected, and productive ways. Their insight, passion, and commitment to the project of queering fat embodiment is inspiring and powerfully transformative.

From Cat:

I am so grateful to have worked on this collection with Jackie and Sam. They have been amazing co-editors, and I could not have asked for better colleagues to have shared my first experience with an edited collection. I am in awe of the contributions we received for this book; the opportunity to work with the authors within these pages is the reason I cherish academia. Their work is strong and insightful; a meaningful contribution to the growing literature of fat studies.

A huge thank you is due to Vanessa Painter, her work in pulling together the details and front/back material was a great help to us all. And thanks are given to Gabrielle Beacham, Spencer Christopher, and my parents for supporting me throughout this process.

Lastly, I'd like to acknowledge the woman who guided me throughout my academic path, and whose lessons and philosophies still guide me today. Without Gwen Sorell, I would not be the scholar or feminist or activist that I am today.

From Jackie:

My first and most profound thanks to my co-editors, Cat Pausé and Sam Murray, who so generously shared their knowledge, experience, ideas, support, and encouragement. Without you, this book would not exist.

To my fat queer community and co-conspiritors, who sustain and nourish me — Aquaporko — Kate James, Georgia Laughton, Moya Carol, Sara Jane Smith, Leonie Bennet, Zoe Holmes, Erin Van Krimpen, Katie Creelman and all the other Porkos — you keep me from drowning. Va Va Boombah – Aimee Rhodes, Lisa Skye and all the other Boombahs and co-conspirators. Jonathan Williams and Isabelle Basher– for many productive conversations about queer embodiment. Katie Chown, for loving me so well for so long. Jenny Lee, for inspiration and patience. Kelli Jean Drinkwater, for fat femme fierceness. Sam Jensen, for endless patience. Emily Turner, for always believing. And all the activists and scholars who paved the way. This collection is for everyone who lives and loves with complicated bodies and desires.

Chapter 1
Introduction:
Why Queering Fat Embodiment?

Jackie Wykes

Queer (and) Fat

Is fat queer? The specious stereotype of the fat lesbian who 'turns to women' because she's 'too ugly to get a man' suggests it may be. Conversely, even the most cursory analysis of contemporary Western media culture reveals that only slender bodies are presented as legitimate objects of heterosexual desire.

These brief examples begin to make apparent some of the ways in which compulsory heterosexuality and compulsory thinness are mutually constitutive. This concept is particularly indebted to Robert McRuer's *Crip Theory* (2006), which in turn draws on Adrienne Rich's 'Compulsory Heterosexuality and Lesbian Existence' (1980). Rich's seminal essay showed how heterosexuality is 'a political institution' which not only works to structure social, political, economic and cultural life according to an asymmetrical system of binary gender, but also how it structures identity and desire through 'control of consciousness'. McCruer drew on Rich's insights to suggest, further, the ways that 'compulsory heterosexuality is contingent on compulsory able-bodiedness, and vice versa' (2006: 2).[1] This collection aims to build on these ideas by examining how compulsory heteronormativity works to regulate fat bodies and subjects, and how this regulation might be challenged through fat scholarship and activism.

Of course, fat scholarship and fat activism are not necessarily distinct categories. Indeed, many of the contributors to this collection straddle the boundaries of academic and activist worlds, as do the editors. Even leaving aside individual personal investments (which are present – if not always explicitly acknowledged – across all areas of scholarship, identity-based or not), fat studies often has the explicit aim of changing the ways that (fat) people – including the scholars themselves – feel and think about, and act

---

1 Several scholars have pointed out parallels between the construction of fatness and disability – and indeed, the ways that fatness is constructed *as* a disability – in contemporary Western culture. For further discussion, see Meleo-Erwin in this volume.

toward, (their own) fat bodies, and thus could be considered a form of activism in and of itself.

The genesis of fat studies as a scholarly field can be traced back to the fat liberation movement that emerged in the US in the late 1960s and early 1970s, growing out of the civil rights and, especially, the women's liberation movements. Early fat activists formed fat women's consciousness-raising and problem-solving groups to address the specific needs and problems faced by fat women, which mainstream feminism often ignored or was even hostile to.[2] These groups later evolved into fat activist collectives such as the Fat Liberation Front and the Fat Underground, and developed insightful critiques of the connections between women's oppression, fat oppression, the medicalisation of the fat body, and the interests of capital vis-à-vis the multimillion dollar dieting and body-modification industries. The Fat Liberation Front also published and distributed these ideas via pamphlets, many of which are collected in the anthology *Shadow on a Tightrope: Writings by Women on Fat Oppression* (Schoenfielder and Weiser 1983). The insights and critiques developed by these early activists groups continue to inform fat activism and scholarship today.

Fat studies as an institutional area of academic enquiry began to emerge in the late 1990s and early 2000s. While a few non-academic books concerning fat politics had appeared before that time (Schoenfielder and Weiser 1983, Millman 1980), fat studies as an identifiable – albeit interdisciplinary – scholarly field developed out of two key contexts: 1) the advent of the 'obesity epidemic' in public discourse; and 2) the material turn in cultural studies, specifically the turn toward 'the body' as an important site for interrogating the operations of power.

The idea of the 'obesity epidemic' began to emerge in public discourse in the late 1990s. While the idea that the general population was getting fatter had already been around for several decades, the late 1990s saw the advent of fatness as a 'global epidemic' and a subject of mediated anxiety. Charlotte Cooper argues that the 'fuzzy origins of what has come to be known as the global obesity epidemic' were 'crystallised' by the World Health Organisation at a summit titled *Obesity: Preventing and Managing the Global Epidemic* (1997) and in the subsequent release in 2000 of a report by the same name (Cooper 2010: 1022).

The construction of fatness as a global health crisis worked to produced fat bodies and fat subjects as both 'diseased' on an individual level, and as parasitic on a social level, monopolising healthcare resources while failing – or refusing – their responsibility as good neoliberal citizens to enact 'proper' self-management through weight loss. Fatness was thus constructed as moral failing (see, for example, the UK House of Commons report on obesity, which

---

2 See, for example, mainstream feminism's embrace of Susie Orbach's *Fat is a Feminist Issue*.

asks 'should obesity be blamed on gluttony, sloth, or both?' (HoC 2004, 23)). As Samantha Murray argues, the discourse of the 'obesity epidemic' not only 'mobilised the moral panic that surrounds an epidemic as an urgent imperative for citizens to lose weight' (2008: 20–21), but produced a rationale for fatphobia in the name of "health" and, moreover, worked to make fat bodies into targets for increased monitoring, surveillance, and intervention.

Meanwhile, feminist and queer scholarship was turning toward the problem of the body, and, in particular, theories of embodiment that emphasised the material specificity of the corporal body in the construction of sexuality and subjectivity (Butler 1990, 1993, Grosz 1994). However, fatness was largely elided in scholarship on the body prior to the emergence of fat studies. Even in work that explicitly engaged with 'embodied difference' or 'subversive' bodies, fatness was rarely mentioned, and the question of fat subjectivity and identity was almost never addressed.

Even more curious was the lack of engagement with fatness in both popular and academic texts that specifically addressed questions of weight. Prior to the emergence of fat studies, several decades of feminist work had analysed the constructions and constrictions of the female body in Western culture (Orbach 1978, Chernin 1981, Bordo 1993, Wolf 1990). Much of this analysis examined body size and weight, but was typically centred on eating disorders and 'the tyranny of slenderness' (Chernin 1981).

While this work yielded valuable insights into the construction of (female) bodies and compulsory thinness that informed, and in some ways enabled, the emergent field of fat studies, it persistently centred on a normatively slender body, marginalising or erasing fat bodies except as the constitutive and often invisible 'other' against which the norm was defined. As LeBesco argues, this focuses on compulsory thinness 'excludes the fat-identified subject' and acknowledges only 'a subject whose desire to be "normal" determines her identity' (2004: 16). Fat studies, in response, has positioned the materially fat body at the centre of inquiry.

Queering Fat

The potential queerness – and queer potential – of fat has long been an important part of the political project of fat activism and scholarship. For example, Kathleen LeBesco's foundational work draws out a number of similarities/ parallels in the medical, psychological, social, and representational treatments of fatness and queerness (2001, 2004, 2009). LeBesco argues that both fatness and queerness are, or have been, medicalised, pathologised, and stigmatised. Both are – or have been – at the centre of moral panics in which they are conceived of as perverse, excessive, unnatural, and a threat to the social order.

Both have been targeted by public health campaigns and other interventions that seek to manage, 'cure', or eliminate them. These discourses produce fat and queer bodies (and fat queer bodies) as 'unfit' both physically and morally.

Importantly, however, 'queer' is not simply a way of describing 'same sex' desire or object choice (even if we leave aside for a moment the problematic concept of 'same sex' with its binary assumptions and neat alignment of sex and gender). Rather, queer can be either (or both) a description *and* an action; an orientation *and* a practice; a mode of political and critical inquiry which seeks to expose taken-for granted assumptions, trouble neat categories, and unfix the supposedly fixed alignment of bodies, gender, desire and identities. As Eve Kosofky Sedgwick argued:

> "queer" can refer to: the open mesh of possibilities, gaps, overlaps, dissonances and resonances, lapses and excesses of meaning when the constituent elements of anyone's gender, of anyone's sexuality aren't made (or *can't* be made) to signify monolithically. (1993: 8)

Sedgwick goes on to suggest that 'a lot of the most exciting work around "queer" spins the term outward along dimensions that can't be subsumed under gender and sexuality at all [such as] race, ethnicity, postcolonial nationality' (1993: 8–9). However, she also cautions against disavowing the originary meaning of 'queer' to denote 'same-sex sexual object choice' since 'for anyone to disavow those meanings, or to displace them from the term's definitional centre, would be to dematerialise the possibility of queerness itself' (Sedgwick 1993: 8).

Questions of sexuality are always implicated in questions of the body, since 'any account of embodiment is also always an account of sexuality' (Grosz 1994: viii). Indeed, as many of the pieces in this collection show, body shape and size are profoundly implicated in questions of gender and sexuality, often in ways that are far more complex and intimate than the conventional discourses of 'body image' and 'self-esteem' can allow.

The pieces in this collection do not simply draw parallels between fat and queer experiences, investigate the intersection of fat *and* queer, or even argue that fat necessarily *is* queer (although these ideas are explored). Rather, the chapters in this collection point to the ways that heteronormativity operates as a regulatory apparatus which underwrites and governs the discourse on – and management of – the fat body.

Furthermore, fatness cuts across lines of gender, sexual orientation, class, race, and ability. While these 'identity-constituting, identity-fracturing discourses' many not necessarily be *subsumed* under gender and sexuality, they are, however, mutually implicated in the discursive and material construction and circulation of meaning, identity, and power that fall under the critical rubric of queer critique.[3] Importantly, 'identity-constituting' discourses such as heterosexuality, able-bodiedness, whiteness, middle-classness and slimness are unmarked – they appear natural and universal and thus have a profoundly normative and disciplinary power. By 'bringing forth' these discourses and making their hidden assumptions visible, queering can work to destabilise normative categories and denaturalise dominant ways of seeing, doing, and being.

Fat identity is not contiguous with any one category (although body size and shape may cluster according to structural factors such as income and ethnicity), but rather intersects with different vectors of identity in mutually constitutive ways. Indeed, as Elena Levy Navarro argues in the introduction to *Historicizing Fat in Anglo-American Culture*, fat has often been understood as a natural, universal, and trans-historical category, thus obscuring 'how fat as a classification serves to secure power relations' (2010: 2). This is not to suggest that fat somehow negates or overdetermines other categories, but rather to emphasise how anti-fat rhetoric is deployed in ways that reinscribe and naturalise extant social inequalities in and through the body (see also Metzl 2010).

This approach moves toward an understanding of the multiple and intersecting ways that power operates on bodies and desires. Importantly, it also points towards the ways in which non-normative bodies challenge and disrupt – that is to say, queer – the disciplinary power of normative categories.

Queering Fat Embodiment

While queer theory has long been influential in fat studies scholarship, this is the first collection of work focused specifically on the critical and political potential of queering fat embodiment. The chapters collected here take a range of approaches to queering fat embodiment, exploring the multiple and overlapping connections and intersections between fat and gender, sexuality and desire, fat embodiment and trans embodiment, fashion and consumption, visuality and art, gay masculinities, neoliberal capitalism, disciplinary medicine, disability, and fat activist politics.

Given the identity-effects/personal investments/etc., it is unsurprising that many of the pieces in this collection are deeply informed by lived experience. As Longhurst notes in this volume, 'the process of constructing knowledge is always embodied'. A number of the papers collected here explicitly acknowledge this when they use personal stories to explicate theoretical arguments. At the

---

3 See, for example, Mason Stokes' *The Colour of Sex* (2001), which examines the ways that whiteness is central to the construction of normative heterosexuality; and while Stevi Jackson's 'Heterosexual Hierarchies' (2011), which explores the interrelations of class and sexuality.

same time, Longhurst argues, '[o]ur subjectivities are made and remade through our research'. This recalls the inextricability of the relationship between fat activism and scholarship – the pieces in this collection seek to bring about transformation, both for the researcher and the reader.

Similarly, James Burford and Sam Orchard's dialogically structured 'Chubby Boys with Strap-Ons: Queering Fat Transmasculine Embodiment' not only draws on the authors' personal experience, but presents 'a co-constructed conversation'. The authors create a deliberately 'messy text' which aims to 'resist dichotomous thinking by proliferating different, and indeed divergent accounts. As they note, '[w]orking in this way frees us as authors to disagree with each other, and ourselves' Burford and Orchard extend this queer approach to knowledge production to the process of reception and meaning-making in the practice of reading, explicitly inviting readers to speak the text aloud, to pay attention to the affective experience of reading, and to speak back.

The pieces in this collection are exploratory and questioning; they suggest ways of thinking about fat embodiment that are contingent, contextual, and relational; they are ruminations and provocations rather than definitive theories or answers. They question orthodox ideas about fatness from both mainstream culture and from within fat studies itself. This volume contains reflective personal narratives, autoethnographic theorisations, and formal scholarship, bringing together different genres and modes of inquiry into the queer potential of fat embodiment. Queering is, after all, interested in troubling the distinctions between categories, and by refusing 'proper' divisions, we hope to encourage productive reflection and connections across and between the collection and its readers.

In the opening chapter, 'Queering Body Shape and Size', Robyn Longhurst outlines four possible approaches to queering fat embodiment: Judith Butler's work on performativity; Michael Brown's work of the closet; Elspeth Probyn's rethinking of shame as an important and potentially productive emotion; and Sara Ahmed's theorisation of the embodied spatial aspects of 'orientation'. In outlining these approaches, Longhurst is seeking to 'un-fix' fatness 'by exposing the fluid and spatially contingent nature of these subjectivities'. Her analysis is informed by her own experiences changing weight as well as her theoretical commitments.

Longhurst's attempts to un-fix fatness challenges one of the orthodoxies of fat politics – that is, that body size is largely beyond individual control. In response to the idea that fatness results from a failure of will, fat activists and critical obesity scholars have argued that body size is more or less fixed, an immutable fact of genetics (see, for example, Campos 2004). This biological determinism may be an understandable response to stigma, but, as LeBesco has argued elsewhere, it is both predicated on a lack of agency, and works to reinscribe the underlying logic which posits fat bodies and subjects as inferior and out-of-control (LeBesco 2004: 114). By 'un-fixing' fatness, Longhurst's work promises to 'open up psychological, discursive and material spaces' for 'a diverse range of perpetually shifting corporeal forms'.

Kimberley Dark's chapter, 'Becoming Travolta', illustrates the queer potential of un-fixing fatness, reflecting on the complexities of fat embodiment, gender, sexuality and identity. Dark tells the story of how, as pre-adolescent girls, she and her friends repeatedly enacted scenes from *Grease*, reflecting on how her fatness meant she was always assigned the role of Travolta – 'I was the biggest of the group, therefore the most convincing guy. Or maybe I was the least convincing Sandra Dee'. Working through the performance to the performative, Dark's narrative shows not only how the specificity of the fat body circumscribes what sorts of (gendered and sexual) roles are available to – and intelligible for – fat girls, but how the continual reiteration of these roles works to materialise sex and gender in and through the body.

Dark illuminates the ways that fatness works to put particular forms of femininity 'out of reach', but suggests that 'becoming Travolta' doesn't necessarily preclude being Olivia: 'for me, the role of male lead AND the female glamour were imprinted utterly'. Rather than negating the possibility of femininity, Dark suggests that fat embodiment can open up the queer potential of sexuality and gender.

Stefanie Jones's chapter, 'The Performance of Fat: The Spectre Outside the House of Desire' spins Butler's performative analytic out along multiple axes of race, class, and sexuality to argue that 'the regulation of fat … is integral to the maintenance of other systems of differentially distributed power' while at the same time 'the construction of fat is informed by systems of race, class, and sexuality and the desire associated with them'.

Jones argues that desire is central to the apparatus of neoliberal capitalism, arguing that the 'threat' posed by fatness is the threat of exclusion from heterodesire and the dominant order. Highlighting the slipperiness of 'fat' as a signifier, Jones argues that 'because it can be used to critique any imagined difference from the social ideal, there are few on whose bodies the term will not stick'. Fatness, then, is deployed as a regulatory category that induces subjects to undertake the 'uncompensated, unending work of individualist self-improvement [which] is a condition of both the body and of labor under neoliberal capitalism'. The persistence of the fat body in the face of this regulatory apparatus 'stands against a simple dichotomy of desire and satisfaction of that desire'.

While Jones recognises that 'fat embodiment twists up and complicates the binaries of heteronormative desire in such a way that can easily be claimed as queer', she argues for a utopian understanding of queer as shifting and contingent. A 'truly queer' fat embodiment, then, would not prefer 'a certain formation of desire', but rather (re)create 'a dynamic of desire that works actively against the processes of heteropatriarchal white-supremacist (and … ablist) capitalism'.

LeBesco's 'On Fatness and Fluidity' also challenges to the supposed fixity of the fat body. LeBesco draws out the parallels between fat embodiment and trans embodiment in order to rethink the possible meanings of intentional weigh loss as a practice of body modification. She argues that dominant narratives construct both weight loss and transition as a permanent, unidirectional move from one side of a binary identity to the other, and proposes the concept of 'sizef*cking' as an alternative possibility with the potential to destabilise binary categories.

LeBesco cautions against an uncritical celebration of an abstracted fluidity which embraces trans and genderqueer as purely theoretical models and ignores the lived reality of embodied subjects. Not only would such a move risk implicitly devaluing 'inflexible' subjects, but it 'disregard[s] both hegemonic constraints on gender diversity in public interactions and the disruptive effect of transgressive fluidity not on the gender order, but on individual lives'.

In 'Chubby Boys with Strap-Ons: Queering Fat Transmasculine Embodiment', Jamie Burford and Sam Orchard interrogate their own experiences of fat and trans embodiment via 'a conversation between two people who (at the time of writing) shelter under the broad trans* umbrella, and focus on accounts of fat embodiment in trans* cultural work'. Their text constructs a complex and contingent network of relations between body size, gender, and desire as they reflect on their ongoing negotiation of identity and embodiment in relation to romantic and sexual relationships, queer communities, biomedical authority, media outlets, self-representation, and more.

They insist on the social embededness of the embodied self, and articulate the ambivalence of being fat and trans in a fat phobic and transphobic world. At the same time, they discuss the productive and enabling possibilities of queering fat transmasculine embodiment by 'proliferating alternative, and (to some) incoherent images and accounts of masculinities'.

Cat Pausé's chapter, 'Causing a Commotion: Queering Fat in Cyberspace', also speaks to the potential of proliferating alternatives to enable new ways of thinking about fatness. Pausé looks at online fat activism, arguing that the Internet opens up new possibilities for building fat community across spatial and temporal disjunctures. She presents a series of case studies that demonstrate the potential for online activists to queer normative ideas about fatness through the refusal of mainstream discourses of health, beauty, and desire, and the creation and dissemination of new ideas about fat bodies and identities.

Jenny Lee's memoir piece, 'Flaunting Fat: Sex with the Lights On', also reflects on the enabling possibilities of fat (and) queer community while exploring the social, cultural, and familial imperatives which delineate fat and queer identities.

Lee talks about 'coming out' both as fat and queer, and suggests that, by denying bodily appetite, dieting serves to keep the fat body 'in the closet'. In particular, her reflections on the connections and divergences between her desire to modify her body through weight loss and her partner's desire to undertake gender transition illuminate the constitutive relationship between body size and gender, specifically the imperative for women to be thin – while 'his desire for change included shedding other people's expectations that he would conform to his allocated female gender and upbringing, whereas my desire for change was about conforming to what I thought a woman should be'. Lee's identification as fat/queer in the closing section of her piece serves to underscore how understandings of body size, sexuality and gender are mutually constructed.

Zoë Meleo-Erwin's 'Queering the Linkages and Divergences: The Relationship between Fatness and Disability and the Hope for a Liveable World' moves from the discussion of gender and onto disability. She traces the medical, cultural and material connections and disconnections in the construction of fatness and (as) disability, and outlines the ways that fat scholars and activists have used the 'social model' of disability to argue that fat subjects are 'disabled' by 'the ways in which the social and built environment create barriers for those with impairments by reflecting and privileging the able-bodied'. While acknowledging the value of the social model in enabling 'the development of a social and political identity, the creation of community, and the opening up of employment, education, community based housing, transportation, access to more of the built environment, etc.', Meleo-Erwin argues that it ultimately rests on neoliberal ideologies which enforce 'normative ideals of autonomy, control, self-determination, and proper citizenship'.

Rather than arguing that fat bodies should be considered disabled, she suggests that fat (and) disabled bodies belong under the umbrella of queer. In making this argument, Meleo-Erwin calls for an examination of how 'concepts such as health, illness, normalcy, pathology, and cure are ideological' and function as normative categories of regulation and control. Queering the construction of fatness and disability, she argues, 'makes room for counter-notions that allow for difference, interdependence, and even vulnerability and choice' and thus create 'the hope of liveable worlds'.

Shifting back to a more explicit focus on gender and sexuality, Scott Beattie's 'Bear Arts Naked: Queer Activism and the Fat Male Body' considers the queer potential of eroticised images of 'the hairy bear body' to disrupt normative ideas of masculinity, health and desire by 'blur[ing] the boundaries of techniques representing masculine and feminine through depiction of hardness and softness, muscle and fat'.

Through a series of interviews with 'bear artists', many of whom identified as straight women, and most of whom 'denied any overt political agenda [and] had little if any connection the bear subculture', Beattie problematises notions of artistic production, authenticity, essentialist identity, subcultural formation, and the politics of activism, arguing that '[b]ear arts can be understood as an aesthetic and discursive force rather than a social and political one without diluting its power to effect change'.

Finally, Margitte Kristjannson's chapter, 'Fashion's "Forgotten Woman": How Fat Bodies Queer Fashion and Consumption', analyses the complex relationships between fatness, femininity, class, taste and consumption. Following Bourdieu, she argues that notions of taste operate as both aesthetic and moral imperatives that are materialised in and through the body and its habits. Given the dominant cultural logic which posits fat people as 'out of control' consumers who 'will eat or buy anything', the logics of taste and consumption work to naturalise not only distaste for fatness, but the unequal social and cultural structures which produce the fat body.

Kristjannson's exploration of fashion also illuminates the ways that access to commodities governs access to social identity and cultural capital. Quoting Sedgwick, she argues that fat women's lack of access to fashion constitutes the 'primal denial' of subjectivity under capitalism: 'there's nothing here for you to spend your money on'.[4]

The chapters in this collection, while wide-ranging in topic and approach, share a commitment to denaturalising received ideas about fatness, even within fat studies itself, and fat activism in its various materialisations and manifestations.

Queering Fat Embodiment, then, is not only a means of inquiring into the ways that bodies and desires are regulated through the system of compulsory heterosexuality, but an exploration of the potential of fat bodies to disrupt normative imperatives and stable categories in broader ways. As LeBesco argues, 'corpulence carries a whole new weight as a subversive cultural practice that calls into question received notions about health, beauty, and nature' (2004: 1–2). By assembling the chapters in this book, we hope to and explore the productive potential of fat to denaturalise ideas about health, sexuality, desire, and embodiment (among others), and build on the productive possibilities of queer (and) fat as both descriptions and actions – to queer fat embodiment, and fatten queer theory. Above all, we hope to provoke further examination of not only the potential queerness of fat, but the queer potential of fatness.

---

4 Sedgwick goes on to explain that 'distinct from the anxiety of never enough money … this is instead the precipitation of one's very body as a kind of cul-de-sac block or clot in the circulation of economic value' (Moon and Sedgwick 2001: 294).

References

Bordo, S. 1993. *Unbearable Weight: Feminism, Western Culture, and the Body*. Berkeley, University of California Press.

Braziel, J.E. and LeBesco, K. 2001. *Bodies Out of Bounds: Fatness and Transgression*. Berkeley, University of California Press.

Butler, J. 1990. *Gender Trouble: Feminism and the Subversion of Identity*. New York, Routledge.

Butler, J. 1993. *Bodies That Matter: On the Discursive Limits of 'Sex'*. New York, Routledge.

Campos, P. 2004. *The Obesity Myth: Why America's Obsession With Weight is Hazardous to Your Health*. New York, Gotham Books.

Chernin, K. 1981. *The Obsession: Reflections on the Tyranny of Slenderness*. New York, Harper.

Cooper, C. 2010. Fat Studies: Mapping the Field. *Sociology Compass*, 4, 1020–1034.

Grosz, E.A. 1994. *Volatile Bodies: Toward a Corporeal Feminism*. St Leonards, Allen & Unwin.

House of Commons Health Committee. 2004. *Obesity*.

Jackson, S. 2011. Heterosexual heirarchies: A commentary on class and sexuality. *Sexualities*, 14, 12–20.

LeBesco, K. 2001. Queering Fat Bodies/Politics. In J.E. Braziel and K. LeBesco, *Bodies Out Of Bounds: Fatness and Transgression*. Berkeley, University of California Press, 74–87.

LeBesco, K. 2004. *Revolting Bodies? The Struggle to Redefine Fat Identity*. Amherst & Boston, University of Massachusetts Press.

LeBesco, K. 2009. Quest for a Cause: The Fat Gene, the Gay Gene, and the New Eugenics. In Rothblum, E. and Solovay, S., *Fat Studies Reader*. New York and London, New York University Press.

Levy-Navarro, E. 2010. *Historicizing Fat in Anglo-American Culture*. Columbus, The Ohio State University Press.

McRuer, R. 2006. *Crip Theory: Cultural Signs of Queerness and Disability*. New York and London, New York University Press.

Metzl, J.M. 2010. Introduction: Why 'Against Health'? In Metzl, J.M. and Kirkland, A. (eds) 2010. *Against Health: How Health Became the New Morality*. New York and London, New York University Press.

Millman, M. 1980. *Such a Pretty Face: Being Fat in America*. New York and London, W.W. Norton & Company.

Murray, S. 2008. *The 'Fat' Female Body*. Basingstoke and New York, Palgrave Macmillan.

Orbach, S. 1978. *Fat Is a Feminist Issue*. London, Arrow Books.

Rich, A. 1980. Compulsory Heterosexuality and Lesbian Existence. *Signs*, 5, 631–660.

Sedgwick, E.K. 1993. *Tendencies*. Durham, Duke University Press.

Shcoenfieldere, L. and Wieser, B. (eds) 1983. *Shadow on a Tightrope: Writings by Women on Fat Oppression*. San Francisco, Aunt Lute Book Company.

Stokes, M. 2001. *The Colour of Sex: Whiteness, Heterosexuality, and the Fictions of White Supremacy*. Durham and London, Duke University Press.

White, F.R. 2012. Fat, Queer, Dead: 'Obesity' and the Death Drive. *Somatechnics*, 2, 1–17.

Wolf, N. 1990. *The Beauty Myth*. London, Chatto & Windus.

World Health Organisation. 2000. *Obesity: Preventing and Managing the Global Epidemic*. WHO Technical Report Series.

Chapter 2

Queering Body Size and Shape: Performativity, the Closet, Shame and Orientation

Robyn Longhurst

Introduction

Queer theory provides a useful platform from which to critique not only heteronormativity (Sullivan 2003, Browne 2006) but also body size and shape. Queer scholars and activists over the past two decades have engaged in a project that aims to queer, trouble or make strange taken for granted sexed, sexual and gendered practices. But it is also possible to queer other practices that tend largely to go unquestioned, such as the desirability (in Western contexts) of being tall and slim. In other words, in the same way that it is possible to 'un-fix' sex, sexuality and gender, by exposing the fluid and spatially contingent nature of these subjectivities it is also possible to 'un-fix' body size and shape. By un-fixing or queering I don't mean simply inserting non-normative body sizes and shapes into the mix but rather that body size and shape are disciplined by social institutions and practices that normalise and naturalise just one type of body and shape over and above others. Natalie Oswin (2008: 90) makes the point that new scholarship in queer studies 'merges postcolonial and critical race theory with queer theory to bring questions of race, colonialism, geopolitics, migration, globalization and nationalism to the fore in an area of study previously trained too narrowly on sexuality and gender'. In this chapter I add body size and shape to this list.

Like sex, sexuality, gender, and race, body size and shape are often treated as material 'things' that are secure and constant; yet as we age, become ill, pregnant, menopausal, change our daily habits, diet, change jobs, recreate, slim, 'bulk up', 'work out', undergo surgery, and shift in and out of various social and spatial contexts, our bodies change in size and shape. To date, there has been some work (but not a lot) both inside and outside the academy that queers fat embodiment (e.g. see many of the contributions in Braziel and LeBesco 2001, especially LeBesco 2001, Martin 2006, Branlangingam's blog 'The queer fat femme guide to life', and Cat Pausé's radio show 'Friend of Marilyn' which 'un-fixes' body size). The aim of this chapter then, is to consider exactly what aspects of queer theory might be most useful for informing critical studies of body size and shape, including but not only fat bodies, in relation to space and place. Trained in the discipline of human geography, I have developed a keen sense of how place and space 'matter' to embodied subjectivity, especially in relation to sex, sexuality, gender (see Johnston and Longhurst 2010) and body size and shape (see Longhurst 2005). The facets of queer theory that I focus on therefore reflect that they offer a route to thinking spatially about these issues.

In the first section I pursue Judith Butler's (1990) notion of performativity. People perform, repeat, and reiterate norms surrounding their body size and shape which then take on the appearance of the natural. Following this, in the second section, I focus on geographer Michael Brown's (2000) work on the closet. While the materiality of body size and shape might seem somewhat obvious and more difficult to closet than other axes of subjectivity, many of the bodily practices associated with body size and shape such as desiring sex with someone who is large, and weighing the body numerous times a day, are often hidden. In the third section, I examine Elspeth Probyn's (2005) contribution on shame and pride. Probyn does not analyse shame and pride as though they are easily separable binary categories treating shame as negative and pride as positive, but instead asks what might be the potentially productive effects of shame. It is not always possible to simply turn shame into pride. Structural relations cannot be ignored. Examining in more depth the politics around shame and pride in relation to body size and shape might be a fruitful avenue for fat studies scholars and activists. In the fourth and final section, I turn to Sara Ahmed's (2006) research on queer phenomenology and what it means for bodies to be 'orientated' or situated in time and space. Many of Ahmed's ideas are applicable to body size and shape because people who are, for example, large, tall, wide, fat, and/or short do not fit comfortably – discursively or materiality – into everyday spaces. Each of these different dimensions of queer theory – performativity, the closet, shame, and orientation – is discussed in turn.

Finally, it is worth noting that throughout the chapter given that the process of constructing knowledge is always embodied (Grosz 1993, 1994), I draw on my own experiences, both personally and of research I've conducted to date, to elucidate the theoretical points being made and to situate myself in the work. Our subjectivities are made and remade through our research. As Gillian Rose (1997: 316) notes, the 'researcher, researched and research make each other; research and selves [are] "interactive texts"'. Research and researchers are not easily separable. This doesn't mean that we can all assume to unproblematically know and represent ourselves but some reflection on our own complex and shifting embodiment can help materialise the notion that our subjectivities are gendered, sexual, that our skin is a particular colour, and that we are a particular body size and shape. These things cannot be easily separated out from our roles as researchers.

Body Size and Shape as Performative

Butler, in her influential book *Gender Trouble* (1990, also see Butler 1993, 2004), problematises the distinction often made between sex and gender. Sexed bodies, Butler argues, cannot be understood as separate from gendered bodies; rather the apparent existence of sex prior to discourse and culture is merely an effect of the functioning of gender. Likewise, the materiality of differently sized and shaped bodies cannot be separated from the ways in which bodies are culturally constructed. It is possible to argue, therefore, that body size and shape are performative and as a result can be troubled. Butler (1993) emphasises the role of repetition in performativity, making use of Jacque Derrida's theory of iterability – a regularised and constrained repetition of norms. This repetition, Butler argues, is not performed *by* a subject; rather it is what enables a subject and constitutes the spatial and temporal condition for the subject.

Over the years I have researched from a feminist poststructuralist geographical perspective gender, sex and sexuality but also fat bodies and slimmed bodies. Years of thinking about both these subjects and my own subjectivity have resulted in me feeling as though I perform my body size and shape just as much as I perform my sex and gender, that is, I repeat or reiterate norms surrounding my body size and shape. I have not necessarily done this consciously but subjects are influenced by societal expectations and culturally imposed values that surround what it means to be a particular body size and shape. I was the fat woman – feminist – who appeared comfortable with her size. I argued with passion about the 'tyranny of slenderness' (Chernin 1983) and refused to abide by the norms constituting feminine beauty. Other body types often accompanied by stereotypical behaviours are the fat man who is jovial, the muscular jock who is athletic but not particularly academic, the skinny teenage boy who is gawky and not quite in control of his limbs, and the thin rich woman who projects an air of superiority. Societal expectations can prompt particular repeated behaviours in sized and shaped subjects that reinforce and/or sometimes contest – or trouble – stereotypes such as these.

Some researchers in critical scholarship on body size are shape and already using this approach of bodies as performative. A useful example that springs to mind is Trudy Cain's (2011) research on 10 self-identified fat women in Aotearoa New Zealand who negotiate the boundaries of their bodies and clothes in particular spaces. Cain does not draw heavily on Butler (but rather on de Certeau 1984), however, she appears deeply interested in the performativities of her participants' lived experiences. Cain asked her participants to keep clothing journals, rummage through their wardrobes with her, take photographs, and allow her to go with them when they shopped for clothes. She focuses on two dominant discourses of fatness: fat as abject; and fat as medicalised. Fat bodies, Cain argues, are performed in particular ways in relation to these discourses. They function to marginalise larger women but larger women also resist, often in quite creative ways, in order to manage (especially through the use of clothing) the marginalisation of their fat bodies.

Rachel Colls' (2007) research on 'Materialising bodily matter' also illustrates how body size and shape are performative. Unlike Cain, Colls does draw specifically on Butler (1993) and aims to extend the notion of performativity by focusing on matter, the material and materialisation (she does this via the work of a range of theorists, especially Karen Barad 2003). Colls argues that performativity needs to grant not only language and culture agency and historicity but also matter itself needs to be understood as having productive capacities. Performative bodies are discursive but constantly lived through their materiality in particular times and spaces. In this way, matter is materialised, it is dynamic. Colls (2007: 358) explores this idea in relation to fat. Fat, she says 'is ambiguous; placed simultaneously under the skin yet materialised as a substance in and of itself'. In short, Colls encourages an understanding of fat as performative but also as 'intra-active' (a term she borrows from Barad 2003, meaning that matter is not passive but an active agent).

These are just two examples that illustrate that Butler's ideas about performativity and iterability are useful not just for understanding sex and gender but also body shape and size in that they provide a way of thinking about the materiality of bodies (e.g. their clothes, flesh, folds) and their mutually constituted relationship with social, cultural and spatial environments at particular times.

By way of a more personal example, throughout my life I have been a variety of sizes and shapes. I have been fat. I've been slim. My body has been firm, and at other times saggy. My adult weight has varied by more than 40 kilos (or 88 pounds or 6 stone). This change in size and shape is not just the result of so-called yo-yo dieting (binging and starving, which I have at times engaged in), but rather reflects various life phases, times, spaces and places: in my early 20s long periods of exhausting international travel – backpacking accompanied by giardia, diarrhoea; loss of appetite; in my 30s, of pregnancy, breast-feeding, lack of sleep, snatching high calorie foods during a busy day; and more recently (over the past couple of years) a 35 kilo weight loss from dieting. I know what it feels like – viscerally and emotionally – to perform a 'normal' body and I know what it feels like to perform a fat body. I have experienced first-hand the privileges and the marginalisation of being different sizes and shapes. For me, different body sizes and shapes have undoubtedly been performative rather than natural, fixed or stable.

Closets and Coming Out

Like performativity, the concept of the closet can also be useful for thinking through the size and shape of bodies. Michael Brown (2000) argues: 'the closet is not just a metaphor for the concealment, erasure, or ignorance of gays' sexualities but it also has a materiality and exists at a variety of spatial scales, from the body to the globe. In the first instance the closet might seem like a surprising area of queer studies to draw on for thinking through body size and shape because bodies, their mass, form, and shape, are visible. Unlike queer bodies, fat bodies, thin bodies, tall bodies or bodies considered to be ill-proportioned in some way, are already 'out'. Clothing is sometimes used to try and alter the look of bodies, for example, undergarments that firm and trim, belts to highlight waists, and wide shoulders to add bulk or make a body appear 'in proportion', but nevertheless the overall size and shape of the body is reasonably evident (see Pausé 2012, and Saguy and Ward 2011 on 'coming out as fat').

What is less visible, though, are some of the eating, exercising, purging and surgical practices that surround the fleshly materiality of the body. Binging, compulsive exercising, using laxatives in an attempt to lose weight, constant weighing of foods and the self, calorie counting, measuring body parts, calculating Body Mass Index (see Evans and Colls 2009) – these things often remain closeted. In relation to my own experiences, sometimes I concealed hurt and shame about my body size, the folds, the chaffing and the sweating. I did not want others to know that I couldn't find clothes that fitted even though I knew this was more about societal norms and the way capitalism functions than it was about me. I sometimes attempted to hide health conditions commonly associated with non-normative bodies (such as back pain caused by large breasts), and I often did not want to admit being subject to comment, ridicule, or sometimes even worse, being ignored on account of being fat. I remained closeted.

Connected to the notion of the closet, I think there is a possibility for arguing the case for more autobiographical or autoethnographic work on body size and shape (e.g. Cooper 2012, Longhurst 2012, Murray 2005, 2010, Throsby 2008). The more that people expose, share, and reflect on experiences of body size and shape, the more it becomes possible to realise that these experiences are wide-ranging, complex and often contradictory. Samantha Murray's insightful reflections on the tensions between her feminist and fat studies scholarship (2005) and her decision to undergo weight loss surgery (2010) is a useful example of the value of this kind of work. I acknowledge that such research, however, can open researchers up to criticism and hurtful comments. For example, when I submitted a manuscript based on autoethnography to a journal reflecting on my experiences of weight loss one of the reviewers wrote:

'Longhurst [the reviewer identified me even though no author name appeared on or in the paper] should shelve this submission and return to it in a few years' time, and then she might have a more realistic and critical piece on the widely shared meaning of weight-loss and likely weight gain … Play the game if you want in your private life, but, in a feminist journal I think contributors need also ask who put the rigged one armed bandit in the room at this historical juncture and who does it most benefit?' (the reviewer is referring here I think to 'the game' of weight loss, that it's rigged in that the diet companies win, that the status quo of revering the slim body is maintained). I am well used to critical comment from reviewers but this reviewer seems to make it personal – perhaps a response prompted by my making the personal public in the first instance. Coming out of the closet then, has both benefits and costs. Sharing experiences of fatness, and in the case of the aforementioned paper, of weight loss, can open up emotional and affectual territory that sometimes prompts empathy and a shared understanding, but other times not.

Another point worth raising about the metaphor of the closet and of coming out is that, as Brown argues (2000: 147), 'People can be in and out of the closet simultaneously … Its space can reveal and conceal at the same time, often dependent on one's own location' (Brown 2000: 147). Diana Fuss (1991) makes a similar point explaining that the difficulty with the inside/outside rhetoric associated with the closet is that it disguises the fact that many people are both inside and outside simultaneously. For example, currently I am slim but still *feel* fat and know that a future self is likely to be fat again. I struggle on a daily basis to limit my calorie intake. In a sense I feel both inside and outside of the closet. Sometimes I disclose these things, other times I do not. Eve Kosofsky Sedgwick makes the point that 'there can be few gay people … however fortunate in the support of their immediate communities, in whose lives the closet is not still a shaping presence' (1990: 68, also see Sedgwick 1993). The same can be said for fat people. Even those who value visibility and the sharing of information openly, at times chose not to disclose.

Those associated with people whose bodies are considered to be non-normative may also at times occupy the closet, for example, so called chubby chasers (heterosexual men who are sexually attracted to large women), or men who are attracted to 'bears' (heavy-set, often hirsute men). Fear of discrimination means individuals may 'come out' about some issues in some contexts but not in others. The closet then can be a useful metaphor for understanding a variety of different embodied subjectivities that people, for one reason or another, might feel troubled about disclosing. Research on fatness that is informed by a liberalism, a politics of equality of sorts that focuses on including fat bodies, does not go far enough in explaining fat people's experiences. Therefore, looking for others ways, such as employing the metaphor of the closet, to try and examine issues to do with body size and space is important.

Shame and Pride

Thinking about closets (both metaphorical and material) inevitably provokes thinking about shame and pride, which are also deeply entangled in the politics of body size and shape. Elspeth Probyn's research, particularly *Blush: Faces of Shame* (2005: 4) offers a route for considering in more depth these concepts. Probyn begins *Blush* stating that she wants to use shame to:

> nudge readers to question their assumptions about the workings of our bodies and their relations to thinking; about the nature of emotions in daily life and in academic reflection; and about ways of writing and relating.

Probyn's main argument is that 'something about shame is terribly important. By denying or denigrating it or trying to eradicate it (as in countless self-help books against various strains of shame), we impoverish ourselves and our attempts to understand human life' (3). Although pride has been an important feature of many new social movements (e.g. gay pride, black pride and more recently fat pride), shame has been virtually ignored, even though, as Probyn argues, it carries with it potentially productive effects. Tracing some of the manifestations or 'faces' of shame, whether they be personal or collective, Probyn suggests, can enable people to reassess their actions, themselves and, importantly, their politics. In these ways, shame, she argues, can be productive.

Jamie Burford (2012), in a paper titled 'Que(e)rying fat pride', reflects on his experiences at the intersections of gay, genderqueer/trans and fat politics in Aotearoa New Zealand paying particular attention to his experience of fat shame and pride in the sexuality and gender diverse communities in which he participates. Shame and pride are locked together in a sense. Another example of work which recognises the mutually constitutive relationship between shame and pride is Samantha Murray's (2008) chapter 'Fattening up Foucault: A "fat" counter-aesthetic?' Murray (2008) engages with Foucault's later work on the 'care of the self' presented in *The History of Sexuality Volume II*, explaining: 'Foucault references the Greco-Roman world when he explains that to live a "beautiful life", one must avoid regimes of excess, and practice control in all aspects of one's existence' (Murray 2008: 125). For Foucault, creating oneself as a 'work of art' was an ethical project. He argues that 'aesthetics of existence' offer enabling possibilities. Murray (2008: 126), however, makes the point that aesthetics are 'not something spontaneously produced in a vacuum by the individual'; rather, aesthetics are learned discursively.

Bodies deemed to be fat tend to be read in most Western cultures as greedy, excessive and lacking in control; therefore for a 'fat' woman to conform to the aesthetic ideals that lie at the core of an 'aesthetics of existence', she would have to radically change her body in order to be seen as 'beautiful'. Murray asks, therefore, 'how much choice does an individual really have in deciding what kind of a subject they want to be?' Surely they are determined within particular sets of discursive relations which cannot simply be deconstructed. One cannot just step outside of these structural relations that constitute the 'beautiful' body, nor can one simply decide to step away from shame and turn it into pride, because subjects are *subject to* the judgements of others. The self does not exist in isolation.

Organisations such as the National Association to Advance Fat Acceptance (NAAFA) have made efforts to change societal attitudes towards fatness by arguing that large people ought not feel shame but instead be proud of who they are, including their size. While it is possible to appreciate this position as a political strategy I think it would be useful for organisations such as NAAFA to engage with some of these more complex ideas about shame and pride as being mutually constituted and entangled at the scale of both the individual and the social. Using Probyn's work to examine some of the discourses of pride and shame that surround body size and shape could therefore be useful.

Probyn herself has already done this, although only briefly, in relation to eating practices by including her own experiences of being 'severely anorexic as a child' (Probyn, 2000: 125). She recalls her 'prominent set of ribs, and pelvic bones that stood in stark relief, causing shadows to fall on a perfectly concave stomach'. Probyn (2000: 125) says looking back at her experiences she wonders 'at the forces of pride and shame doing battle in a body that knows itself to be disgusting'. Her memories are 'tinged with a mixture of shame, disgust and guilt' (Probyn, 2000: 125). I think these ideas about pride and shame are interesting and could be teased out further in relation to body size and shape.

Queer Phenomenology

Sara Ahmed, in her book *Queer Phenomenology: Orientations, Objects, Others* (2006), focuses on the 'orientation' aspect of 'sexual orientation'. Interestingly for me as a geographer, Ahmed examines what it means for bodies to be situated in space and time. She argues that bodies take shape as they move through the spaces directing themselves toward or away from objects and others. Ahmed's insights on 'lived experience, the intentionality of consciousness, the significance of nearness or what is ready-to-hand, the role of repeated and habitual actions in shaping bodies and worlds' (2006: 2) are invaluable for thinking about body size and shape. Being 'orientated' means feeling at home, knowing where one stands, or having certain objects within reach. Orientations affect what is proximate to the body or what can be reached.

While Ahmed pays attention to queer orientations, these ideas are also applicable to bodies in relation to size and shape. For example, people who are large, tall, wide, fat or short. often do not fit comfortably into various spaces and places encountered in daily lives. The objects they encounter do not function to make the person concerned feel comfortable or orientated. For example, interviews I conducted with large women (Longhurst 2010), and my own experience, indicate that chairs are often too flimsy for large-bodied people, inbuilt seats are too narrow, retail clothing store changing rooms are too small, clothes are not cut and sewn to fit large bodies comfortably, images of bodies that are meant to be attractive are nearly always of slim, taut bodies. Social relations (in this instance, a privileging of bodies that fit within a very narrow range of heights and weights) are constituted spatially, discursively and phenomenologically.

One particular participant, Denise, in the aforementioned study (Longhurst 2010) illustrates this point about some bodies not fitting. Denise is 1.9 metres (6 feet 2 inches) tall and has large feet. She finds it difficult to find shoes that fit. Denise also finds shopping for clothes challenging and explains: 'I just feel stupid. They are all size 8 and I am size 20. Then if you go to the big women's clothes they cater for women that are my height but really really big so you get the tent dresses' (Longhurst 2010: 207). Denise avoids shopping for clothes as much as possible. She often feels 'disorientated' in everyday spaces, whether they be shops, beaches or pubs. At beaches Denise does not like to wear a swimsuit, at pubs she often gets 'hassled'. She says that she wishes she could live her life in big spaces, and if she ever got to design her own home 'it would be big house ... I would like to design a house with a tall toilet. I would like a tall toilet and my friends can have a step and I am quite happy with that ... I need lots of space. It's not my idea of fun being in small spaces' (Longhurst 2010: 210).

Other participants in the same study, including Sandra and Miranda, also reported feeling that they do not fit comfortably into everyday spaces on account of their body size and shape. Sandra says: 'I don't fit well into airplane seats anymore, or hairdressers. I used to go to a salon but I couldn't fit into their waiting seats. Coffee lounges, some of their seats are too small' (Longhurst 2010: 210). Miranda, aged in her mid 40s, does not like the seats at rugby matches because you have to sit in an allocated, joined seat which is 'really little ... actually tiny'. Miranda says the seats at her local theatre are also 'really tiny' and that she feels like she is 'exploding' on to someone else's seat, which makes her feel very self-conscious.

Ahmed argues that queerness disrupts and reorders these relations of proximity by not following accepted paths; so too does having a body that does not confirm to a normative size and shape. Ahmed (2004: 1) says: 'Bodies take the shape of the very contact they have with objects and others' and that 'Comfort is the effect of bodies being able to 'sink' into spaces' (Ahmed 2004: 152). People whose bodies do not fit the norm on account of their shape and size are rarely comfortable sinking into their surrounding spaces because these spaces are not constructed to fit their bodies.

Conclusion

Jagose (1996: 16) argues: 'heterosexuality is too often represented as unremarkable' and as the normative position from which other sexual identities are seen as derivative. Following this line of thought it can also be argued that slimmed bodies are too often represented as the unremarked norm from which other body shapes and sizes are seen a derivative – fatter or thinner than the norm, taller or shorter than the norm, and so on. Although queer studies has mainly be used as a platform from which to critique heteronormativity, Sedgwick (1993) claims it can also be applied to a broader range of normative knowledges and identities than just sexual ones. She explains:

> a lot of the most exciting work around "queer" spins the term outward along dimensions that can't be subsumed under gender and sexuality at all: the ways that race, ethnicity, postcolonial nationality criss-cross with these *and other* identity-constituting, identity-fracturing discourses, for example. (Sedgwick 1993: 8–9, italics in original)

One could add to this list body size and shape. Fiona Giles (2004: 303) notes that there is likely to be some resistance to queering something that is not usually perceived to be overtly sexual but it is evident that 'queering can usefully be applied to any behaviour that is extravagantly regulated'.

Body size and shape and the practices that surround them are undoubtedly highly regulated. Perhaps it is not surprising therefore that queer studies has a great deal to offer scholars and activists in fat studies and critical geographies of body size and shape. For example, it is able to provide a fertile space for interdisciplinary engagements. As scholars and activists we have different educational backgrounds, disciplinary training, and preferred ways of working, but these differences can be productive for queering our conversations on a variety of topics including body size and shape. These conversations do not represent one-way relationships and ideas and once transferred from one disciplinary area to another would not remain unchanged. For example, fat studies and critical geographies of body size and shape may offer up just as many important insights to those in queer studies as queer studies may be able to offer up to those in fat studies and critical geographies of body size and shape.

It is important to remember, however, that queer studies is not a uniform body of work and some threads may be more productive than others for scholars and activists focusing on body size and shape. I have chosen to examine just four threads – performativity, closets, shame and pride, and queer phenomenology – but I am sure there are others that some are already using to inform research which are equally if not better suited for thinking through body size and shape. Finally, then, queer studies offers possibilities for 'un-fixing' body size and shape which has potentially liberating effects. Queering body size and shape – that is, understanding and accepting a diverse range of perpetually shifting corporeal forms – can open up psychological, discursive and material space for appreciating a wider range of bodies than just a select few.

References

Ahmed, S. 2004. *The Cultural Politics of Emotion.* New York: Routledge.

Ahmed, S. 2006. *Queer Phenomenology: Orientations, Objects, Others.* Durham and London: Duke University Press.

Barad, K. 2003. Posthumanist performativity: Toward an understanding of how matter comes to matter. *Signs: Journal of Women in Culture and Society,* 28(3), 801–831.

Branlandingham, B. 2013. The queer fat femme guide to life. [Online, 22 February] Available at: http://queerfatfemme.com/ [accessed 22 February 2013].

Braziel, J.E. and LeBesco, K. 2001. *Bodies Out of Bounds: Fatness and Transgression.* Berkeley: University of California Press.

Brown, M. 2000. *Closet Space: Geographies of Metaphor from the Body to the Globe.* London: Routledge.

Browne, K. 2006. Challenging queer geographies. *Antipode,* 38, 885–893.

Burford, J. 2012. Que(e)rying fat pride. Paper presented at 'Fat Studies: Reflective Intersections', 5 July 2012. Massey University, Wellington Campus, New Zealand.

Butler, J. 1990. *Gender Trouble: Feminism and the Subversion of Identity.* New York: Routledge.

Butler, J. 1993. *Bodies That Matter: On the Discursive Limits of 'Sex'.* New York: Routledge.

Butler, J. 2004. *Undoing Gender.* New York: Routledge.

Cain, T. 2011. Bounded bodies: The everyday clothing practices of larger women. PhD thesis (Sociology, Massey University, Albany, New Zealand).

Chernin, K. 1983. *Womansize: The Tyranny of Slenderness*. London: The Woman's Press.

Colls, R. 2007. Materialising bodily matter: Intra-action and the embodiment of 'fat'. *Geoforum*, 38(2), 353–365.

Cooper, C.R.M. 2012. Fat activism: A queer autoethnography. PhD (University of Limerick, Ireland).

de Certeau, M. 1984. *The Practice of Everyday Life* (S. Rendall, trans.). California: University of California Press.

Evans, B. and Colls, R. 2009. Measuring fatness, governing bodies: The spatialities of the Body Mass Index (BMI) in anti-obesity politics. *Antipode*, 41(5), 1051–1083.

Fuss, D. 1991. *Inside/Out: Lesbian Theories, Gay Theories*. New York: Routledge.

Giles, F. 2004. 'Relational, and strange': A preliminary foray into a project to queer breastfeeding. *Australian Feminist Studies*, 19(45), 302–315.

Grosz, E. 1993. Bodies and knowledges: Feminism and the crisis of reason, in *Feminist Epistemologies*, edited by L. Alcoff and E. Potter. New York: Routledge, 187–215.

Grosz, E. 1994. *Volatile Bodies: Toward a Corporeal Feminism*. St Leonards: Allen & Unwin.

Jagose, A. 1996. *Queer Theory*. Carlton, Vic: Melbourne University Press.

Johnston, L. and Longhurst, R. 2010. *Space, Place, and Sex: Geographies of Sexualities*. Lanham: Roman & Littlefield.

LeBesco, K. 2001. Queering fat bodies/politics, in *Bodies Out of Bounds: Fatness and Transgression*, edited by J.E. Braziel and K. LeBesco. Berkeley: University of California Press, 74–87.

Longhurst, R. 2005. Fat bodies: Developing geographical research agendas. *Progress in Human Geography*, 29(3), 247–259.

Longhurst, R. 2010. The disabling affects of fat: The emotional and material geographies of some women who live in Hamilton, New Zealand, in *Towards Enabling Geographies: 'Disabled' Bodies and Minds in Society and Space*, edited by E. Hall, V. Chouinard and R. Wilton. Farnham: Ashgate, 199–216.

Longhurst, R. 2012. Becoming smaller: Autobiographical spaces of weight loss. *Antipode: A Radical Journal of Geography*, 44(3), 655–662.

Martin, F. 2006. Queer intersections: Sexuality and gender in migration studies. *International Migration Review*, 40, 224–249.

Murray, S. 2005. Doing politics or selling out? Living the fat body. *Women's Studies*, 34(3), 265–277.

Murray, S. 2008. *The 'Fat' Female Body*. Basingstoke: Palgrave Macmillan.

Murray, S. 2010. Women under/in control? Embodying eating after gastric banding. *Radical Psychology*. [Online] 8(1) Available at: http://www.radical psychology.org/vol8-1/murray.html [accessed 25 February 2013].

Oswin, N. 2008. Critical geographies and the uses of sexuality: Deconstructing queer space. *Progress in Human Geography*, 32, 89–103.

Pausé, C. 2012. Live to tell: Coming out as fat. *Somatechnics*, 2(1), 42–56.

Pausé, C. 2013. Friend of Marilyn Show on Access Manawatu Community Radio. [Online, 20 March] Available at: http://www.accessradio.org/public/ programme.php?uid=1313540452-463-11 and http://friendofmarilyn.com/ [accessed 20 March 2013].

Probyn, E. 2000. *Carnal Appetites: FoodSexIdentities*. London: Routledge.

Probyn, E. 2005. *Blush: Faces of Shame*. Minneapolis: University of Minnesota Press.

Rose, G. 1997. Situating knowledges: Positionality, reflexivities and other tactics. *Progress in Human Geography*, 21(3), 305–332.

Saguy, A.C. and Ward, A. 2011. Coming out as fat: Rethinking stigma. *Social Psychology Quarterly*, 74(1), 53–75.

Sedgwick, E.K. 1990. *Epistemology of the Closet*. Berkeley: University of California Press.

Sedgwick, E.K. 1993. *Tendencies*. Durham: Duke University Press.

Sullivan, N. 2003. *A Critical Introduction to Queer Theory*. Armidale: Circa, 43–44.

Throsby, K. 2008. 'Happy re-birthday: Weight loss surgery and the "new me"'. *Body & Society*, 14(1), 117–133.

Chapter 3
Becoming Travolta

Kimberly Dark

Saturday Night Fever was the first R-rated movie I ever saw. I sat uncomfortably next to my mother during the whole film knowing that, at some point, someone would have sex and she'd have her eye on me.

And there it was: John Travolta and the woman he will dump have sex in the back seat of a car. But I was even more uncomfortable when that young woman cried because Travolta hooked up with someone else. I could feel my mother's smugness. That trollop got her comeuppance. It was her own fault and my mother wanted me to take a lesson. That's what I imagined anyway. Later, at home, as she was ironing and I sat on her bed, my mother wanted to know if I had any questions about such an 'adult film'.

Good heavens no! Under no circumstances did I have any questions about that film. La-la-la. I tuned out whatever she said next. It was awful. The next time I saw an R-rated film with my mother was probably 20 years later, and it was only slightly less uncomfortable.

When I'm a guy, in my mind's eye, I'm a young John Travolta character. I'm Vinnie Barbarino from *Welcome Back Kotter*, or I'm dancing in a white suit in *Saturday Night Fever*. Or better yet, I'm in all black with my hair slicked back, singing, 'You're the One that I Want' in the final scene of *Grease*.

It's not that I'm interested in being a guy, or taking on a romantic role other than my own, but Travolta is part of my adolescent history. He's really the only male actor I've imitated with any regularity – and I became Travolta across a range of characters.

My friends and I loved the music from *Saturday Night Fever*. The Bee Gees were dreamy and the Gibb brothers were the hotness of the day. Andy Gibb performed the first big stadium concert I ever saw. Though the film was important, not all of my friends were allowed to see it – because it was rated R – and the night club bar-scene it depicted was a little complicated and disturbing for some of us. We mostly listened to the music and ignored the film. The romantic dancing was too hard to imitate anyway. We stuck with hip shaking and that diagonal up and down pointing thing that Travolta did in his white suit.

When *Grease* came out a year later, however, we were in our element. It was 1978; my friends and I ranged in age from 10 to 13, and the plot line was easier to understand than *Saturday Night Fever*. There was no urban grit, just the silly suburban setting in which our plot lines were also played, despite the 1950s being long gone. *Grease* was a superbly satisfying love story for us – and what did we love best? The transformation of Sandra Dee.

Wow! We all wanted to be her – to have *that* kind of power over *that* kind of guy. Wow! We loved the greased lightning song, squirmed through 'Hopelessly Devoted' waiting for it to end. But then, over and over, we'd dance and lip-sync and sometimes even sing 'You'd better shape up! 'Cause I need a man, and my heart is set on you ...'

The trouble with the burning need to put on this spectacle over and over again was that we were all girls. Boys had no interest in playing this game (and we'd have likely been embarrassed to ham it up around them anyway). And we ALL wanted to be Sandra Dee in her shiny spandex pants and stiletto heels.

But in my friend group of four, I was always cast as the leading bad-boy greaser. It was my destiny. I already knew the score, and had come to embrace my role in the group. Ask anyone who grew up as a fat girl if she ever got the female lead with thinner girly girls around. I'd put money on the answer being no. This is probably also true for girls who were considered unattractive, if their prettier friends wanted those roles. We didn't even discuss it – that's just the way it was. Someone had to be Travolta and it was going to be me. I was the biggest of the group, therefore the most convincing guy. Or maybe I was the least convincing Sandra Dee. No discussion was needed. We took our roles from Hollywood and did our best to divvy them up and act them out in our child-bodies. You can't try out for just any old part. You won't get it and you'll only humiliate yourself trying.

Of course, it isn't actually true. Some girls learn to be pretty by reading the fashion magazines, using make-up in just the right way. If she's thin, a girl can learn to put on glamour, but that doesn't work as well for fat girls. Glamour was the reason Sandra Dee became a knockout, after all. She was just a pretty little girl before the final transformation. She was just – nice. With her hair all curled up, wearing bright lipstick and stilettos, she became the trophy for which Travolta could openly yearn and compete.

So, I practiced that part where Travolta falls to his knees in front of Olivia Newton John over and over. I practiced the shoulder-leading hunch with which he follows her as she slinks away only to return and dominate him again and again. I sang, 'You're the one that I want' and my other two friends (the Sandra Dee understudies) added in the falsetto 'ooh, ooh, ooh'. I practiced as my bouncy little blonde best friend – herself insecure in her freckled beauty – vamped over me in a silly, theatrical way, wearing her older sister's stiletto heels and ill-fitting spandex pants. The other two girls in our foursome were understudies for Olivia Newton John – sometimes they were hand-on-hip Stockard Channing just for fun. But I was Travolta.

It's not like I hadn't been prepared to take the role that supports feminine stardom. I already knew the score from being excluded from things like gymnastics class and ballet. The teachers wouldn't know what to do with a body like mine and besides, it would just be cruel to put a girl like me in leotards and tights to be laughed at. So I became the spotter when my friends practiced their backbends and walk-over handstands. Literally a supporting role; I knew how to praise their effort, spot good precision and budding talent, though never within myself. (I only learned as an adult, in my own yoga practice, that I could've done those backbends and handstands too.)

I have to admit, I adored being Travolta, though I could never take the role public, in the same way my friend was actually practicing to act like sexy Sandra Dee at parties and dances. I was doomed to be a closet Travolta, never a public Olivia Newton John. So much potential, wasted as a wallflower.

At some point, I started to realise there were more like me: fat girls who could really dance and knew what it meant to be hot – fat girls who knew how to be funny and smart. We were observers and supporters and yet, we were also Travolta – the leading man in our own minds. Though we became with zeal, we didn't stop being Olivia Newton John inside. Though I became Travolta, I remained Olivia. I took on his assuredness, but not his arrogance. I took on his voice, but not his content. I learned how to facilitate others' successes and how to speak up to make a point, but I stopped short of exercising privilege because that vessel was empty. I became Travolta, in the way only a fat girly-girl can. Sure, some girls who grew up to identify with masculinity were probably pleased as punch to become Travolta – never gave Olivia another thought. Those are the women I date – but I wasn't one of those.

I suspect that the masculinising of fat girls, ugly girls, and gay girls can have a fabulous side effect. We learn about assertive femininity. We learn about wearing different gender roles. We learn about living in our bodies and being glamorous when we choose. And for some of us – we do all of those things at once and we grow up to be assertive, fat, femme dykes. There are more than a few of us out there – and I've always wondered how we got to be so fabulous without any role models. It takes some gumption to be other than average in the female category (fat and queer) and to reclaim – and sometimes exaggerate – the big prize that Sandra Dee held aloft in *Grease*: assertive sexy femininity.

Becoming Travolta, as I did, wasn't an entirely raw deal. He was the leading man, after all. My other two friends only understudied Olivia Newton John – we ALL did that – but for me, the role of male lead AND the female glamour were imprinted utterly. And I didn't just become Danny Zuko in *Grease* – I became Travolta. He's had a long and varied career with lots of different roles. Our adolescent experiences stick with us – and I could've done worse. I was lucky enough to become Travolta. Even after I was grown, some part of me still expected the leading man role – after all, I've also two-stepped with Debra

Winger in *Urban Cowboy* and twisted with Uma Thurman in *Pulp Fiction*. And I was Debra. I was Uma.

Romantically, this versatility served me too. When the time came, I knew how to be hot like the leading ladies – but I also knew how to prompt my butch lover to be the best Travolta she could be. I knew it because I lived it. I didn't want to take that role, but I did it until I didn't have to anymore. Armed with Travolta-skill, I know how to prompt it in others. And for the girls who only ever wanted to be Travolta, I am a beautiful homecoming. Some of my lovers have been grateful that I showed them, in my way, how to get comfortable as the male lead. And my butch lovers return the favour; they are women who know how to appreciate femininity, but they also know how to read and prompt my complexities.

Sure, it'd be a better world if we all had the freedom to be all the characters we liked best – one by one and in innovative combinations. I hope that day is coming. And becoming Travolta wasn't so bad. It's amazing how the roles we didn't want can make us richer sometimes.

Chapter 4

The Performance of Fat: The Spectre Outside the House of Desire

Stefanie A. Jones

Introduction

The construction of material bodies is not just biological. It is a necessarily social process. Judith Butler states in the introduction to *Bodies That Matter* (1993):

> what constitutes the fixity of the body, its contours, its movements, will be fully material, but materiality will be rethought as the effect of power, as power's most productive effect. ... Once "sex" itself is understood in its normativity, the materiality of the body will not be thinkable apart from the materialization of that regulatory norm. "Sex" is, thus, not simply what one has, or a static description of what one is: it will be one of the norms by which the "one" becomes viable at all, that which qualifies a body for life within the domain of cultural intelligibility. (2)

In short, the social audience's reception (via constructed categories) of sex make the body possible. Similarly, this chapter explores the categorisation of fat embodiment. Tensions around the 'fat' body reveal its status as a particular kind of sign that makes classed, sexualised, and racialised bodies, and as signifier that amplifies that (dis)connection between material bodies and heteronormative, white-supremacist capitalist desire. A relational exploration of 'fat' performance within debates about class, sexuality and race highlights the contradictions inherent in the idea of bodily fixity and strengthens Butler's argument that the 'material' body (as much as gender) is itself a construction of discourse.

This chapter begins with an examination of various frameworks for understanding fat embodiment. It explores the need to move away from quotidian understandings of 'fat' and phenomenological understandings of 'embodiment' towards a (necessarily social) performance understanding of fat embodiment. This social frame is well-elucidated by a relational exploration of the meaning of fat embodiment. The relational social reception of performances of fat helps us understand the manifesting materiality of bodies as receptors or resisters of capitalist, racist, and heteronormative desires.

I then go on to explore the way that structures of class, sexuality, and race play with and around negotiations over desire and fat bodies in performance. This investigation reveals the importance of desire and bodies to neoliberalism. It also exposes certain elements of how bodies function under neoliberalism, particularly bodily self-regulation and uncompensated disavowed labour. Throughout I attempt to illuminate negotiations over fat bodies and desire, and how those negotiations make and are made by bodies.

This exploration also reveals that fat embodiment, while defined by dominant power hierarchies, presents a potentially political limit to the dominant modes of power within such hierarchies. This break is queer in the sense that it is opposed to or destabilising of binary constructions of desire. The fat body stands against a simple dichotomy of desire and satisfaction of that desire. But this formation of queer itself isn't necessarily political; it could be as much used to challenge the status quo as to work for conservative ends. Finally, I propose a pre-ontological politics that could serve as the beginnings of a truly queer fat embodiment.

Performance: Understanding Fat, Understanding Embodiment

In the quotidian world, even those whose bodies literally serve to define the thin ideal can be marked as fat. As the social ideal arises out of social images (and with decreased funding to the arts in the United States, for example, most of our social images are media and advertising images populated by positive depictions of the bodily 1 per cent), perhaps nothing represents this so well as the shrinking of the ideal body within the fashion industry. For example, Trebay (2010) in the popular press reports on model Coco Rocha, whose modelling work has all but disappeared because, at a size 4, she is considered too fat. Categorising someone as fat can be completely disconnected from biological markers; the meaning of 'fat' itself is destabilised.

Here mere formal linguistic understandings of fat embodiment fail us. Cooper (2010) provides excellent intellectual and political justifications for using the term 'fat' over other terms that are used to engage with the discourses of fat studies. Cooper finds 'fat' studies as a field to be a critical and social method for understanding bodies that terms such as 'obesity' cannot capture, and the former to be more free from and critical of the moralising and pathologising implications of the latter. Even considering these justifications, Cooper's overview of the field acknowledges (but doesn't fully engage with the idea) that the sign 'fat' is itself complex. The signified indicates a variety of different body shapes and sizes, and the signified is indicated by a variety of different signifiers. In fact, its very variety makes the sign itself suspicious; further investigation reveals that the term is incredibly slippery. 'Fat' can be pinned to so many bodies that the signified it indicates clearly exists outside of physical determinants. Indeed, the term 'fat' pushes the limits of definitional boundaries in its looseness; because it can be used to critique any imagined difference from the social ideal, there are few on whose bodies the term will not stick.

Although not unique to the sign 'fat', such slipperiness indicates an area of contestation in the field of symbolic power. Bourdieu (1999) defines symbolic power as: 'a power of constructing reality, and one which tends to establish a *gnoseological* order: the immediate meaning of the world (and in particular of the social world) depends on what Durkheim calls *logical conformism* (166, emphases in original). This logical conformism is a kind of common sense of things that permits different minds to agree or at least to communicate. The realities constructed by symbolic power are granted legitimacy by 'public expression and collective recognition' (129), and the power of those who constructed these realities is reinforced in the process. So, symbolic power is a way to create the meaning of the world, to which groups agree and conform in public and recognise collectively, and in which process the creators of meaning affirm their power in that position. The *field* of symbolic power, then, involves negotiations over legitimacy, 'a struggle over ... the power to impose (or even inculcate) the arbitrary instruments of knowledge and expression (taxonomies) of social reality – but instruments whose arbitrary nature is not realized as such' (168). This is the power to determine collective, social meaning. Signs in which the signified and signifier are so loosely connected seem to be particularly pointed places to investigate the social forces struggling over this field of symbolic power.

The sign 'fat' exerts authority; when used on bodies it has the power to irrevocably mark people with or without the consent or participation of that person. But it is noteworthy that the flexibility of the term only extends to its expansion to include *more* bodies; contraction to exclude them is much more rigid. Put another way, in current social manifestations in the West, bodies can enter into the sign 'fat', but they may not necessarily be able to escape. For example, to insult someone by calling them fat works as an almost unimpeachable sully. The person insulted cannot deny it, nor defend against it rationally (that is, using evidence), because the body itself, no matter its size, serves as counter evidence that works against such claims. The social use of the term 'fat', then, does something. Instead of the statement of fact that it appears to be, a statement such as 'you are fat' in this sense is performative. Austin (1962) defines the performative as a statement that, instead of indicating something that is true or false, is part of doing an action. Related to or as a consequence of the meaninglessness of the sign, calling someone fat, indeed, *thinking* of someone as fat is constative (a sub-category of the performative for Austin): it makes them so.

The performative is only one example of a fat performance dynamic, and a particularly powered one at that. Performance itself is always at least two-sided: there must be some kind of performer, and some kind of audience. In the description of the performative use of fat above, we can consider the 'fat' person the performer, and the person doing the describing as the audience (although it is clear that there are many different permutations in which the audience is also performer and the performer also some kind of audience, let's stick with this simpler model for understanding an individual within a larger social context for the moment). We have already begun to explore how the audience has significant symbolic power in the described performative dynamic. As I discussed, the audience has the balance of power in the use of the term 'fat', but both sides of the performance dynamic cannot be completely separated. The audience and performer always work to create the meaning of a performance together; while we can acknowledge that the power imbalance lies in the audience's favour, the fat performer is never totally powerless. How do the performers in this equation interact with and influence such a strong audience response? As performance is always defined by both the intentions of the performer and the ideas/needs of the audience, the performance of the fat performer (the enactor of fat embodiment) might be better understood in such an unevenly-powered dynamic as a 'performcemance'. The (fat) body is, by the force of circumstances, necessarily performing as a fat body. While the fat performer still has the quotidian agency to act in a plethora of ways, the audience's intentions are so weighty in determining the actual meaning of the performance that the performer's work is necessarily an enactment of those audience expectations. Indeed, although fat is a social construction (that is, a body's designation as fat is relative, mutable, and assigned by external forces), bodies marked as fat also cannot escape such a classification. The only way to avoid this classification is for the gaze to bounce off, for the namer to decide otherwise. Thus the (fat) body is never not at 'risk' for performing fat.

While there are numerous parties who would prefer to cast 'fat' as scientific fact instead of a socially-inflected performance, such discussions leave unexamined the limits of their own positivism. Cooper outlines the work of these scholars: she identifies both proponents of 'dominant obesity discourse' and opponents of this discourse who use the scientific language of obesity and/or chemical energy in their attempts to pin down understandings of fat, to solidify the term. Connecting realism to the positivism at the centre of modern science, Diamond (1997) observes that, 'because it naturalizes the relation between character and actor, setting and world, realism operates in concert with ideology (4). That is, realism is appealing because external appearances seem to reflect internal truths, not just within the realm of the performance, but between the performance and the rest of the world. These internal truths are, in fact, ideological values. Fat as fact permits us to devalue fat bodies and ignore our social complicity in the creation of the meaning of 'fat' as a devalued social group and the consequences of that devaluation. It is exceptionally promising to use fat performance, then, to read against the 'scientific' realist interpretation of fat embodiment, in order to open up the ideologies that are inherent yet obscured in such positivism.

So merely trying to come to terms with the term 'fat' is insufficient because the word comes alive as it is used, and the body is forced into a particular 'realistic' social performance of fat when the concept comes into play. In *Gender Trouble* (1990), Butler provides foundational work in the field of bodies and performance. Also engaging with Austin, Butler explores the phenomenology of gender, finding gender to be performatively constructed from sedimented repetitions of acts. LeBesco expands on this work in the 2001 chapter 'Queering Fat Bodies/Politics', using the intersections of queer theory and performance studies to politically reposition fat identity in the cultural imaginary. However, LeBesco focuses on subject construction and agency (one side of the performance equation) because LeBesco's project engages with identity. Fat is somewhat more similar to sex than gender because of its connection to material bodies (although we've seen that connection is shaky). Fortunately, Butler's 1993 *Bodies That Matter* expands her exploration of phenomenology to what is traditionally understood as biological: sex. Directly referencing Austin's constative performative, in *Bodies That Matter* Butler states that:

> to claim that discourse is formative [of sex] is not to claim that it originates, causes, or exhaustively composes that which it concedes; rather it is to claim that there is no reference to a pure body which is not at the same time a further formation of that body. In this sense, the linguistic capacity to refer to sexed bodies is not denied, but the very meaning of "referentiality" is altered. In philosophical terms, the constative claim is always to some degree performative. (10–11)

In response to reductive readings of *Gender Trouble*, Butler insists on the power of discourse to constitute and delimit the body itself through a careful examination of the interactions between discourse and ontology. It is this understanding of the biological that makes *Bodies That Matter* so much more compelling for me than *Gender Trouble*. Butler's scepticism of the mimetic quality of the process of signification betrays a radical imagination. Butler can demand that we understand sex as constituted by discourse because our world is conceivable without sex. This is not a patriarchal post-sex dystopia in which the sexed femininity is obliterated in favour of a more neutral masculinity, but rather a worldview that sees as possible as wide a range of sexes as can be imagined and put into discourse. By implying a utopian post-sex possibility, Butler resists the ideological limitations of performative realism by accepting something anti-ideological (non-binary biological sexes) as conceptually possible and realistic. Nonetheless, while she can imagine such a potential for sex, she insists that materiality makes demands on discourse, and later affirms some necessary realities of the body, including 'weight' (66).

Why is Butler's approach sufficient for analysing sex but not certain other elements of material bodies? Butler's approach to interpreting identity is phenomenological which, with its focus on the strength of accumulated acts, has the benefit of having space for the possibility of resistance to oppressive structures such as heteronormativity. For all of Butler's emphasis on *performativity* however, phenomenology offers an understanding of predominantly one side of this performance equation: the performer or subject as they come to be in the world. Butler as phenomenologist does recognise the dependence of subject development on discourse, a necessarily social process. However, some theorists attempt to move beyond the first-person in their understanding of embodiment. In her seminal work *The 'Fat' Female Body*, Murray (2008) looks to a more social phenomenology of the body via philosopher Maurice Merleau-Ponty, approaching embodiment as a process of being both 'subjects "in-ourselves", *and* subjects "for-others"' (6, emphasis in original). Such a social interpretation is more appropriate to understanding performative processes.

MacKenzie (2008) faults Butler for her wholly negative understanding of the matter of the subject. In other words, Butler can determine what the matter of the subject is not, but not what it is. MacKenzie claims that Butler finds 'any attempt to attribute positive content to it [as] reify[ing] a contingent formation as pre-political ontology' (np). I don't agree with MacKenzie's disapproval, but rather find the critique to be reflective of a major asset of the post-structuralist approach: an insistence on the primacy of the political over the ontological.[1] Nonetheless, I understand that Butler's use can be turned into a theoretical trap: if nothing can be understood except in negative, then what is the value of inquiry other than deconstruction, and where is there room for change, for attempts to achieve justice?

It is in order to retain this benefit of phenomenology (the pre-eminence of the political) but move beyond its limitations with respect to performance that I suggest a turn to sociologist Pierre Bourdieu's work. Bourdieuian sociology

---

1 This critique is perhaps best articulated by philosopher Susan Buck-Morss in a 2011 interview with the Polish intellectual magazine *Kultura Liberalna*. Buck-Morss says, 'by resolving the question of Being before subsequent political analyses, the latter have no philosophical traction. They are subsumed under the ontological *a priori* that itself remains indifferent to their content ... The only criterion left for accuracy is internal consistency'.

provides a dialectical theory that doesn't neglect attention to the agency of individual subjects but emphasises the shape of power and how fields of power interact with one another. Such an approach offers an opportunity to resist the reification that Butler critiques while simultaneously providing a chance to understand a value of materiality by analysing the material's temporary position within a time- and site-specific but fluid power hierarchy. By looking at the *process* of materialisation of these constructed-by-discourse bodies, we can at least attempt to gain a clearer understanding of the power dynamics of that discourse, of what brings the body into existence. Philosopher G.W.F. Hegel's (1977) concept of *aufhebung* is particularly useful for elucidating the move to sociology.[2] In a way we can understand Bourdieuian sociology as a process that *hebt* post-structuralist understandings of the limitations of discourse *auf*, incorporating the ideas of instability, relationality and performativity while moving beyond the deconstructionist feedback-loop that in its anti-materialism prevents analysis of material consequences.

A focus on the material is especially important for issues of social justice. While a deconstructionist approach might recognise the fluidity and temporality of bodies and the ultimate meaninglessness of the sign 'fat' in order to challenge the sign's power, individuals are clearly affected by the material consequences of anti-fat bias on their quotidian lives. These run the gambit from economic disparities (Rayno 2011) to psychological distress (Myers and Rothblum 2005). These consequences are serious and material, yet not necessarily ontological. The meaning of fat embodiment will be defined in various times and places by its impact on and relation to the other fields of power with which it intersects, providing an enhanced way to understand embodiment by examining the role of fat performance in relationship to other areas of contestation. Understanding fields of struggle in which fat comes in to play, such as race, class, and gender, is central to understanding fat.

Fat Embodiment in Relation

Following Murray's (2008) observations of the spectre of the 'normal' body that is used to connect Western moral understandings of the body to clinical discourse, I am suggesting that fat comes into play by haunting certain performances of power struggle. Since this is a fluid process, a useful analogy is power as a kind of choreography (a pattern of the steps and moves of each performer in a dance, that, when combined, creates the carefully orchestrated

---

2 The most common translation to English is 'sublate' but this is somewhat less evocative than the three contradictory meanings inherent in the German term: to preserve, to negate, and to move beyond.

total picture of the dance as a whole), where the 'dancers' are players in a variety of intersecting fields. Fat performance allows us to visualise those structured routines as proponents of certain fields that stumble through or around fat bodies with varying degrees of anxiety or grace. Just as a critic might judge a dance on its overall beauty and grace, observers of these power struggles have the ability to connect values to the struggle as a whole (what is more 'appropriate', who is more 'deserving', and so on); the audience has a regulative power when it does the act of observing. In this equation, however, power hierarchies are also performed: players of various sizes and statuses have unarguable power to act in their respective fields (to take particular steps), but their limitations reveal the distribution of power within these fields. Examining such interactions in the fields of class, race, and sexuality, the remainder of this question will ask: what actions *are* taken? And which players are able to secure audience support, and thus to control and determine the social meaning of their actions?

Class

To understand struggles over class, let us consider a hypothetical quotidian performance of 'fat': a public lunch where a visibly fat-bodied person orders either a cheeseburger or a salad. Although both provide caloric sustenance for human life, they have the potential to result in very different performances. Cultural associations with the cheeseburger run the gamut from McDonald's to the epicurean; independent of the source, however, the cheeseburger in our performance connotes laziness, lack of self-control, unhealth, and constant indulgence that are commonly associated with fat in contemporary Western culture. Despite these associations, it is nonetheless conceivable that it might take a great amount of work and self-control to acquire even an occasional cheeseburger, and that even the healthiest of people might make such decisions. Conversely, the salad is the symbol of a dieter; it is associated with health, self-respect, and hard work.

These value associations are tied up with the idea of the fat body *and* with the cheeseburger; each association feeds and is fed by the others. Read as a performance of realism, the social and moral worth of a performer at first appears to be defined by the objects with which the performer interacts. These associations partially constitute the fat performance of ordering a cheeseburger: for certain bodies (the thinner limit of which, as I've discussed, becomes difficult to pin down), the act becomes defined by its associations with caloric fat. Causality is assumed. The fat person orders the cheeseburger *because* they are fat. The person is fat *because* they order the cheeseburger. If it is the performer's interactions with objects that define their reception, then interacting with an object that has positive associations with 'health', as indicated by lower caloric fat (such as a green salad), seems like it would decrease negative associations between the performer and health. But a fat body ordering a salad still recollects the uncontrollableness of the fat body, as well the associations of laziness, unhealth, and indulgence. These associations are now placed to read the performance as one of a-realism: the salad is an exception, the salad is somehow a conduit of excess. The associative order becomes one where any concepts of health connected to the salad are actively disconnected from the fat body. The reception of realism falters, or is disrupted. Once again, the performance of the fat person ordering a salad is also partially constituted by the reception of that act as about fatness. The fat person orders the salad *because* they are fat. The person is fat *because* they order the salad. The individual's performative connection with that item is physical and temporary instead of ontological and eternal, replicating the ideology of positivism.

A performative similarity exists independently of the material circumstances of the performance or the ontological nature of the food items. This example is meant to illustrate that *even if* proponents of 'dominant obesity discourse' and others who attempt a scientific definition of fat were correct in their science, scientific explanations themselves fail to fully elucidate the meaning of fat in its social performance. The caloric count of the salad or the cheeseburger that is understood to be the scientific indicator of health is secondary to the social meanings ascribed to the performance. What appears to be indicated by a sign is disconnected from its actual meaning; the 'health' value of food is not part of its nature but arises as a result of its use within a powered field. Such scientifically 'realistic' readings are particularly compelling in light of Diamond's observations about realism.

Numerous studies, such as the early work 'Influence of Social Class on Obesity and Thinness in Children' by Stunkard et al. (1972), have established a close connection between socioeconomic class and body size. As Bourdieu (1984) explores in great depth, in mid-1960s France, class divisions produce and are produced by indicators of taste. Evans (2010) works from Bourdieu to explore the relationship between size, taste, and class. A fat performer's interaction with a cheeseburger or a salad from a fast food restaurant is more likely to resonate with the ideological associations earlier examined as being tied up with the concept of fat. While interactions with a gourmet cheeseburger or salad from a more elitely-marked source such as a high-end restaurant also invokes these problems, reception of such a performance can be dismissed as a result of the rational and independent choice of the consumer. Because it costs more time and money but is seen as a better investment, the performance of consumption is less ontologically constitutive of the performer's body, the result of an excusable rational indulgence that is less related to the base instincts of the person's body. The purported superiority of the product makes it seem less unhealthy to consume. Thus patterns of reception are altered though the body might stay the same; the performance is altered because of a change of setting and prop. Class privilege provides the performer with a greater distance between the body and the valued associations of the item. This distance is sufficient to justify the consumption but not to decouple the act from the body.

At the same time, working-class bodies are expected to be larger because they are perceived as being less in-control through their connection to baseness, naturalness, and labour (LeBesco 2007). Of course, the conditions of capitalism often demand that these bodies remain large both for the physical demands of work and for the economic demands of a broad capitalist consumer base.[3] Because fat bodies are cast as out-of-control, human needs (food, clothing, shelter) are recast as uncontrolled desires; their position as desires provides the moral ground for corporations to profit off of the fulfilment of these needs.

Sex/uality

With objectification as fat often defined in opposition to sexual objectification, performances of fat embodiment and the reactions to those performances also illuminate dynamics of heterosexual desire. This insistence on the *primacy* of bodily value contradicts the purported pleasure and value of the individual in the heteronormative relationship structure. That is, the body becomes a limit point that contradicts hetero feminine narratives such as true love, the soul mate, and the 'he likes me for me' concept of being valued for one's 'true self'. Despite the agency, freedom, and individual worth implied by this discourse on love, one party has the power to decide the other's value, and that value is dependent on that other working to maintain their position of desirability. Their desirability is always partially determined by the body; what follows is a monitoring and regulation of behaviours, preferences, and habits meant to define and shape the body itself. This bodily policing is emphasised by the constant threat of the fat body, and is a fundamental condition of what Berlant and Warner (1998) identify as 'heterosexual culture'. The fat feminine body is particularly important in such a dynamic. Removed from both the symbolic masculine power of defining the desirability of women's bodies, as well as the position of bodily 'superiority' that give 'desirable' women the symbolic

---

3 Here I do not intend to reproduce problematic assumptions that connect body size and consumption. Rather I mean simply to point out the way that the basic human needs of a variety of sizes of human bodies are additionally exploited by monopolised markets, and how this process serves the consolidation of capitalism. At the time of this writing, the plus-size clothing industry in the United States is an excellent example of the way that negative associations with fat lead to a dearth of producers despite market size, which in turn drives price up and quality down. If these bodies were not marked as exceptional, an exceptional (that is, additional) industry would not thrive off of them.

power to define the undesirability of other feminine bodies, the fat feminine body is twice-removed from the dominant position in heteropatriarchal culture. This complete, twice-removed social rejection is distinctly queer (that is, it is structurally external to the heteropatriarchal binary), and in this queerness is both limiting and liberating.

With 'the heterosexual couple … no longer the referent or the privileged example of sexual culture', Berlant and Warner suggest that there is a radical hope for a culture that 'changes possibilities of identity, intelligibility, publics, culture, and sex' (548) to appear. But performances of fatness are always received by audiences who play a role in defining their meanings.[4] No position or action is political *a priori*; whether or not queerness is political depends on its relationship to material, historical circumstances (Puar 2007). Fat embodiment may feel immediately beneficial for the individual, queerly defiant in the face of a social de-sexualisation that comes from the expulsion from the frame of heterodesire, but this power exists in relation to the current arrangement of fields. This very queer power oddly only exists to the extent to which fat bodies are considered undesirable. It is possible to conceive of a world in which, for example, fat bodies are exoticised or normalised, and thus gain cultural capital; they might then serve to validate heteropatriarchal power instead of to work against it.

In the current moment in the Western world, because it is constructed against social devaluation of fat bodies, fat embodiment is a kind of queer power expressed in the face of normative power. Queer fatness, then, is a condition of living the removal from heteronormativity, of working to defy the symbolic power that determines the meaning of one's body from the outside. Necessarily expelled from the paradigm of heteronormativity, the fat body is regulated to the periphery, left in a no-man's land of desire. Although access to the house of the heteromasculine couple is restricted, the body persists creepily, threateningly outside the window. In the heteronormative construction, the spectre exists for the feminine as the ever-present threat that she might become fat, and lose her status in that house. The masculine is menaced even further; the fat body exists as evidence that his power is not irreproachable, that his ability to control the female bodies around him may constantly be challenged by other forceful agents, that the 'sexual universe' is in fact not universal, nor his.

The fat body's persistence threatens the very existence of the heterosexual paradigm of desire: with doors to keep the fat body out and windows through

---

4 For example, on the stage today fat women's performances are received as hypersexualised because it controls their sexual expression as another symptom of their excess, which can be criticised, instead of their right as fully realised human subjects with human desires, which may still be read as impermissible. See for example, 'Chapter Three: Ravenous Women', in Mobley (2010).

which to regulate it, this 'universe' is much smaller than it seems. Other than literal violent intervention such as murder or mutilation, all attempts at bodily control are only sociocultural. The body cannot be eliminated. Outside of violence, the living body cannot be condensed or compacted *without the action of that person*. However, within masculine constructions of appropriate heteronormative behaviour, bodily regulation is a moralised necessity, and rampant.

Race

Negotiations over desire do not just serve to maintain class differences and promote heteronormative bodily regulation. In the US, race, sex and class are deeply entangled, and race and racism are inextricably bound up with body size and desire. Bogle (2004) studies popular representations of black women's bodies to find that they are consistently juxtaposed to an ideal of thin white femininity. Bonilla-Silva (2006) explores the shift from explicit, biology-based racial essentialism to what he terms 'cultural racism'. As explicit racism becomes socially unacceptable to express, any preference for white bodies (sexually, socially, representationally or otherwise) becomes expressed as the preference for unattached attributes (that, as it turns out, continue to predominantly indicate whiteness, whether or not those attributes are actually attached to white or black bodies). Preferences for a purportedly neutral culture (such as preferences for a purportedly deracialised slenderness) come to stand in for preferences of a more socially unacceptable form (such as disapproval of the racialised fat mammy figure in US American culture, see Bogle 2004). Novelist Zadie Smith reveals and critiques the deep connection between fat, race and desire in her 2005 novel *On Beauty*:

> When you are no longer in the sexual universe – when you are too old, or too big, or simply no longer thought of in that way – apparently a whole new range of male reactions to you come into play. One of them is humour. They find you funny. But then, thought Kiki, they were brought up that way, these white American boys; I'm the Aunt Jemima on the cookie boxes of their childhoods, the pair of thick ankles Tom and Jerry played around. Of course they find me funny. (51)

A quick deconstruction reveals that fat and race are inextricably connected. Smith begins in this excerpt with an impersonal discussion of the nature of a specific system of desire. This system is explicitly male, and has clear limits boundaries of containment. But with even only one repetition of the word 'too', Smith intentionally leaves those boundaries in a realm of formal and material uncertainty. We are unsure what excludes you from the 'sexual universe', but that exclusion itself *is* certain. This part of the excerpt is decidedly marked by the use of the second person narrative; it is almost a direct address to the reader or audience, inviting them in to immediately experience exclusion. Beginning with an understanding that existing as sexual for men is not the most important thing in the world, Smith's narrative notes that exclusion from the 'sexual universe' opens up possible modes of being (such as 'humour') in a way that seems promising, almost hopeful. But the next line involves an abrupt closing-off of meaning; it is no longer the potential for mutual humour but instead their humour at you. This shut down of meaning is apparent in the narrative shift; Smith next moves to the first-person embodied by the third-person. By making the speaker specific, Smith makes historical the overarching concept of the 'sexual universe' with a reference to a current form. The excerpt is no longer a rumination on human relations generally, but instead a reflection on the specifics of the life of Smith's fat, black character Kiki, and the reader/audience is oddly expelled from Kiki's exclusion, providing a clearer view of Kiki's world than Kiki has herself. For Kiki, the humour of her reception (what makes her, now, desirable) is intimately about both race and size. They are inextricable. Thus in this quotation the discovery is that masculine behaviour, with respect to fat, manifests in and from particular cultural histories of racist representation. This quote reflects the text's story of white, masculine desire as a whole complex, from which issues of size, race, and sexuality cannot be excised or untangled. Kiki expresses succinctly the violent and total exclusion of fat (and other) bodies from the necessarily white 'sexual universe'. In revealing the way that fat black bodies are expelled or peculiarly included within this universe, we can see that universe more clearly as broadly about desire under majority discourse. Much as we explored in the section above, this majority discourse constitutes desire as primarily sexual desire, but because Kiki is reaccepted as funny it is evident that this is also about the worth of bodies broadly, the conditions necessary for the desire of their presence. As Kiki reveals in this story, a fat black woman's body must labour to provide another kind of desexualised value: in this case, support for racist narratives of entertainment (such as her re-embodying the Aunt Jemima that she describes). Without such labour, exclusion from the universe of desire is complete.

Conclusion

As scholar Oliver (2006) explores, what links representations of blackness, poorness or working-class status, and fatness are that they 'violate some of the most fundamental tenets of American culture: that all people are fundamentally responsible for their own welfare' (72–3), as well as the values of self-control, self-improvement, and restraint as virtues. While Oliver links these to a religious history, he also mentions the role of capitalism. Indeed, extreme individualism is one of the central cultural features of the practice of neoliberalism in America, the moral necessity of free market mentality. With respect to size, this manifests as the obsessive drive for appearance-based self-improvement, regardless of consequence. The ideas that one can and should labour for or purchase alterations of the appearance of one's body (via clothes, make-up, or surgical interventions), and that the inability to meet social standards of appearance is a deep moral failing, are the ultimate expression of individualist market-centrism and are supported by a ripe industry (Oliver 2006, Gaesser 2002). This is the flaw with Berlant's (2007) attempt to theorise the fat body within capitalism in 'Slow Death (Sovereignty, Obesity, Lateral Agency)'. While Berlant's writing on the subject is often compelling, it misses a thorough understanding of the way that *negotiations* over body size (instead of body size itself) are symptoms of the neoliberal world. Those who spend or labour to regulate their body size are as much the atrophied 'subject[s] of capital' (779) and as lacking in 'practical sovereignty' (778) under capitalism as those who do not. Recognising instead that bodies of a variety of sizes have always existed, we must read the fat body not as a symptom of neoliberalism, but instead *note* the *function* of the fat body within neoliberalism. Through comfortably deceptive misconnections (supported by performative realism) between visible form and concepts of consumerism, the symbolic power of the audience in the equation of fat performance is not only harmful to the performers in that equation; the work used to maintain this symbolic power is also used to establish and maintain other hierarchies of oppression. Audiences use their symbolic power over the idea of 'fat' to cast fat bodies as scapegoats, in order to release social and political pressure arising from the malfunctions of heteropatriarchy, white supremacy and late capitalism.

Therefore, the regulation of fat becomes at least a part of a system of exercising bodily control that is integral to the maintenance of other systems of differentially distributed power. Fat is not just used to classify bodies according to race, class and sexuality, but to maintain systematically the categories of differentiation. Simultaneously, the construction of fat is informed by systems of race, class and sexuality and the desire associated with them. Fat and its reception is a tool that stands in for explicitly unacceptable discrimination, a code for the permissible regulation of bodies along dominant-group lines.

Ultimately, then, what we see through negotiations over and around fat, are negotiations of the power of desire in contemporary neoliberalism. Despite the discourse of individualised, inevitable, biological desire in popular use in the United States today to justify initiatives such as the legalisation of gay marriage, comparing relational uses of fat reveals desire as a firmly social construction. Representation serves as a powerful machine in the construction of desire, such as media/marketing images meant to construct the desire for ownership and purchase of a particular good, brand, or lifestyle (Holt 2004).

These operate through a variety of mechanisms, from the explicit use of bodies in advertisements to the appealing narrative of a television show that keeps up the rates of viewership. Such media representations notoriously present slender white heterodesirable bodies as the acceptable norm. Indeed, these inherently social representations do not just show bodies. The best media images construct bodies as, and connect bodies with, both concepts of desire and the product, brand, or idea for sale. The body and the product are combined and enhanced by the performative aural and visual language of marketing, to *create* the desire that marketing wishes to attract (Araujo 2007).

This process of producing desire isn't limited to the media, however: desire under neoliberalism controls the production and regulation of bodies themselves. As Deleuze and Guattari explore in *Anti-Oedipus*, desire produces further production. 'Producing is always something "grafted onto" the product [of production]; and for that reason desiring-production is production of production, just as every machine is a machine connected to another machine' (2000: 6). If slender bodies are marketing's product, the presence of those bodies in excess produces desire for those bodies, and the desire to produce those bodies. The regulation of bodies into the category of 'fat' reveals that group as opposed to (and yet necessary for) the establishment of white patriarchal heteronormative control over the realm of desirability. The latter creates the former as a regulative category, not merely reflecting its symbolic power to create categories and define meanings, but, much more seriously *to promote self-regulation by the objects of desire*. Scholars such as Mobley (2010) use Foucault's theories to examine how the category 'fat' serves to require subjects to struggle to remain outside that category, to labour without compensation to produce the body-regulation that, outside of force, can only be performed by subjects themselves. This uncompensated, unending work of individualist self-improvement is a condition of both the body and of labour under neoliberal capitalism.

Thus fat performances not only function socially as bodily and behavioural regulating devices (for sexuality, race, and class), but they also perform for a disempowered and isolated furious political mass,[5] invested in realism as an attempt to find meaning in the ultimately arbitrary world of late capitalism. Fat performances are performances of failure. Despite the attempts to structure bodily self-regulation, both the consciously and the unintentionally fat disrupt the model that defines bodies as fundamentally objects for a particular kind of desire. Anti-fat hatred is rage about bodies disobeying those rules of desire, rules which promise elusive benefits to those who follow them. Desire for these purported benefits does the affective work of promoting heteropatriarchal

---

5 When I speak of a furious political mass, I am referring to the US audience, but this must also be considered part of a global audience. See, for example, Ferreira da Silva (2007).

white-supremacist neoliberalism; when those impossible desires are less than satisfying, the bodies that break up that perpetual environment of desire are easy targets for the expression of rage. Because the model of body-as-desired-object demands that fat bodies exist literally outside of that universe, these bodies should be eliminated. *And yet these bodies persist.* The production of the 'fat' body by the audience that calls it into being reveals the need for the negative definition against which to set its desiring machine, and this need for the desexualised fat body permits the audience (the social whole) to continue. Indeed, as Deleuze and Guattari explore, 'desiring-machines work only when they break down, and by continually breaking down' (2000: 8). The process that creates this dichotomous opposition (between body-as-desired-object and undesirable) reveals bodily control as not just at the centre of desire, but as the determining factor of desire under neoliberalism.

In this way we can see anti-fat hatred as a glimpse of the weighty but disavowed consequences of neoliberal ideologies of independence, meritocracy, and the free market. This is one of the very markers of struggle over capital: those in positions of authority control the terms of discourse, which are utilised in such a way to obscure the interestedness of those parties. As Swartz (1997) explicates Bourdieu, 'the exercise of power in almost all cases requires some justification or legitimation that creates "misrecognition" of its fundamentally arbitrary character ... the logic of self-interest underlying all practices – particularly those in the cultural domain – is misrecognized as a logic of "disinterest"' (89).

Epilogue: A Note on Queer

For a collection on queering fat embodiment, queerness has been a surprisingly difficult subject to approach in this chapter. Even though the idea came up in the section on sexuality, it was quickly restricted and delimited. But in a way, this whole chapter has been about the limits of a non-queer fat embodiment. While it is clear that fat embodiment twists up and complicates the binaries of heteronormative desire in such a way that can easily be claimed as queer, I tend to conceive of queer as a utopian political term. As I have stated several times in this chapter, and as many others have argued, queer in the sense of gay or non-normative sexuality is not necessarily political. To get at the utopian queer, I return again to Buck-Morss's (2011) understanding of a pre-ontological politics. A truly queer fat embodiment, then, will shift and change with time and circumstances. Currently, a queer fat embodiment will work to meet the need for a radical love that is not based on individualistic neoliberal desire, but instead, on desire informed by political choice and consequence. In this dynamic, queerness is not defined ontologically as preferring a certain formation of desire, but foremost politically: as a dynamic of desire that works actively against the processes of heteropatriarchal white-supremacist (and, unexplored here, ableist) capitalism.

References

Araujo, L. 2007. Markets, market-making and marketing. *Marketing Theory*, 7, 211–226.

Austin, J.L. 1962. *How to Do Things with Words: The William James Lectures delivered at Harvard University in 1955*. New York: Oxford at the Clarendon Press.

Berlant, L. 2007. Slow death (Sovereignty, obesity, lateral agency). *Critical Inquiry*, 33(4), 754–780.

Berlant, L. and Warner, M. 1998. Sex in public. *Critical Inquiry*, 24(2), 547–566.

Bogle, D. 2004. *Toms, Coons, Mulattoes, Mammies, and Bucks: An Interpretive History of Blacks in American Films*. 4th Edition. New York: Continuum Press.

Bonilla-Silva, E. 2006. *Without Racists: Color-Blind Racism and the Persistence of Racial Inequality in the United States*. 2nd Edition. New York: Rowman and Littlefield Publishers, Inc.

Bourdieu, P. 1984. *Distinction: A Social Critique of the Judgment of Taste*, translated by R. Nice. Cambridge, MA: Harvard University Press.

Bourdieu, P. 1999. *Language and Symbolic Power*, translated by G. Raymond and M. Adamson. Cambridge, MA: Harvard University Press.

Buck-Morss, S. 2011. Sometimes to progress means to stop, to pull the emergency brake. *Kultura Liberalna*. [Electronic journal] Available at: http://kulturaliberalna.pl/2011/12/27/sometimes-to-progress-means-to-stop-to-pull-the-emergency-brake/ [accessed 9 September 2012].

Butler, J. 1990. *Gender Trouble: Feminism and the Subversion of Identity*. New York: Routledge.

Butler, J. 1993. *Bodies that Matter: On the Discursive Limits of 'Sex'*. New York: Routledge.

Cooper, C. 2010. Fat Studies: Mapping the field. *Sociology Compass*, 4(12), 1020–1034.

Deleuze, G. and Guattari, F. 2000. *Anti-Oedipus: Capitalism and Schizophrenia*, translated by R. Hurley, M. Seem, and H.R. Lane. Minneapolis, MN: University of Minnesota Press.

Diamond, E. 1997. *Unmaking Mimesis: Essays on Feminism and Theatre*. New York: Routledge.

Evans, A. 2010. Greedy bastards: Fat kids, class war, and the ideology of classlessness, in *Historicizing Fat in Anglo-American Culture*, edited by E. Levy-Navarro. Columbus, OH: Ohio State University Press, 146–176.

Ferreira da Silva, D. 2007. *Toward a Global Idea of Race*. Minneapolis, MN: University of Minnesota Press.

Gaesser, G.A. 2002. *Big Fat Lies: The Truth about your Weight and your Health*. Carlsbad, CA: Gurze.

Hegel, G.W.F. 1977. *The Phenomenology of Spirit*, translated by A.V. Miller. New York: Oxford University Press.

Holt, D. 2004. *How Brands Become Icons: The Principles of Cultural Branding*. Boston, MA: Harvard Business School Press.

LeBesco, K. 2001. Queering fat bodies/politics, in *Bodies Out of Bounds: Fatness and Transgression*, edited by J.E. Braziel and K. LeBesco. Berkeley, CA: University of California Press, 74–87.

LeBesco, K. 2007. Fatness as the embodiment of working-class rhetoric, in *Who Says? Working-Class Rhetoric, Class Consciousness, and Community*, edited by W. DeGenaro. Pittsburgh, PA: University of Pittsburgh Press, 238–254.

MacKenzie, J. 2008. Judith Butler, gender, radical democracy: What's lacking? *Transformations: Journal of Media & Culture*. [Online], 16. Available at: http://www.transformationsjournal.org/journal/issue_16/article_04.shtml [accessed 15 November 2012].

Mobley, J.-S. 2010. *Staging Fat: Dramaturgy, Female Bodies, and Contemporary American Culture*. PhD dissertation, CUNY Graduate Center (3408058). Ann Arbor, MI: ProQuest/UMI.

Murray, S. 2008. *The 'Fat' Female Body*. London: Palgrave Macmillan.

Myers, A.M. and Rothblum, E.D. 2005. Coping with prejudice and discrimination based on weight, in *The Psychology of Prejudice and Discrimination, Revised*, edited by J.L. Chin. Santa Barbara, CA: Praeger, 187–198.

Oliver, J.E. 2006. *Fat Politics: The Real Story behind America's Obesity Epidemic*. New York: Oxford University Press.

Puar, J.K. 2007. *Terrorist Assemblages: Homonationalism in Queer Times*. Durham, NC: Duke University Press.

Rayno, A. 2011. When it comes to salaries, size does matter–body size. *The Washington Post*, 30 January [np]. Available at: http://www.washingtonpost.com/national/when-it-comes-to-salaries-size-does-matter---body-size/2011/01/28/ABTpl9G_story.html [accessed 2 January 2013].

Smith, Z. 2005. *On Beauty*. New York: Penguin Books.

Stunkard, A., d'Aquili, E., Fox, S. and Filion, R. 1972. Influence of social class on obesity and thinness in children. *Journal of the American Medical Association*, 221(6), 579–584.

Swartz, D. 1997. *Culture & Power: The Sociology of Pierre Bourdieu*. Chicago: University of Chicago Press.

Trebay, G. 2010. A Model's Prospects: Slim and None. *New York Times*, 16 February [np]. Available at: http://www.nytimes.com/2010/02/16/fashion/16DIARY.html [accessed 7 December 2011].

Chapter 5
On Fatness and Fluidity:
A Meditation

Kathleen LeBesco

There is strife within the universe of fat activism surrounding the practice of intentional weight loss. This chapter sets out to examine the logic of contested claims about the meaning of the shrinking fat body. It then explores the value of notions of fluidity that are embraced in queer theory, offers words of caution about a wholesale embrace of fluidity, and considers the future of fat politics in light of body ambivalence.

Strife

Fat activism is currently wrestling with an important question: how does the movement make sense of a fat activist who intentionally loses weight? A number of activists want to stigmatise such activity, arguing that pride and acceptance of fatness run directly counter to an impulse to change.

Fat activist Marianne Kirby, who blogs at *The Rotund*, expresses a common sentiment when she writes:

> there is a lot of damage done to the idea that you, as an activist, accept yourself when you are working specifically to lose weight. I hate to say that. I hate to sound in the least bit exclusionary. And I'm not voting to kick anyone out of the Team Fat club. I think people who are trying to lose weight should absolutely be involved in reading fat blogs and talking to people in the size acceptance community. But there is, rightfully so, I feel, a stigma associated with that choice to lose weight. It runs counter to the very idea that fat activists are working so hard to promote: that being fat is not a statement of morality, is not a personal failing, is not a sign that a person doesn't care about their own body or the feelings of those around them. That being fat is, simply, being fat. (2007)

Similarly, Curran Nault argues that 'embodied corpulence is about taking pride in the fat body in its existing state and refusing to change, shrink or disappear' (Nault 2009: 1). The central question posed by fat activists of this stripe is: Why would one willingly change away from something they accepted, or even that they took pride in?

Surgery as the means to weight loss ups the ante on this question. It is possible that changes in eating and movement divorced from an explicit agenda of weight loss that in fact result in weight loss can be read affirmatively by fat activists who endorse the Health At Every Size (HAES) paradigm, which emphasises listening to one's body and practicing excellent self-care. 'While the line between healthy lifestyle choices and dieting might be a fine one, it is usually the rejection of weight loss per se as a means to improve health that separates the two' (Meleo-Erwin 2011: 195). But there is no provision in HAES or mainstream fat acceptance organisations for bariatric surgery, no way in which surgical intervention (even if framed as the remedy for medical ailments rather than a quick ticket to weight loss success) is typically read as anything but dangerously problematic on a number of fronts – the physical, alimentary, and political. Some fat activists describe bariatric procedures as 'mutilation' or 'amputation', 'considering them a medically-mediated and socially-sanctioned form of eugenics and/or genocide against those who are fat' (Pfeffer 2012: 25).

Pinpointing the strife surrounding bariatric surgery, Samantha Murray writes eloquently about the disruptive effects on her body, on her eating practices, and on the way her politics were perceived after pursuing gastric banding. 'While embracing the aims of the fat liberation movement and the varied forms of committed fat political activism that seeks to end discrimination against fat people and to encourage a celebration of size diversity, I also often struggled with feelings of ambivalence about my embodiment' (Murray 2010: 43). She did not want her actions to confirm a general belief that weight loss is essential to health, but she sought a solution for pain and lethargy. Post-surgery, she critiques the very practice that one might see as facilitating her fluidity: 'Surgery merely resituates food and eating as the central aspect of one's existence, and demands the ongoing physiological and psychic exercise of control, thereby disturbingly reaffirming fat bodies as fundamentally *out* of control' (Murray 2010: 52). Elsewhere, of course, Murray encourages fat activists to move beyond the mind-body split and to tolerate body ambivalence (2008).

This embrace of ambivalence is exemplified by others in the fat activist movement who push back against the indictment of intentional weight in the community. Zoë Meleo-Erwin writes about fat activist Hanne Blank, who in 2007 documented her attempts to lose weight in a blog. 'Blank calls attention to what she sees as a hypocritical stance in fat activism wherein those who adopt a HAES approach and "accidentally" lose weight are not demonised within the movement but those who do so consciously are' (Meleo-Erwin 2011: 196). Meleo-Erwin notes that Blank, like Murray, seeks to complicate what she sees as the type of overly 'black or white' stance toward intentional weight loss, epitomised by Kirby, above. 'Further, she sees blanket anti-weight loss stance of fat activism silencing and suggests that pushing the envelope on 'hot button' issues is necessary to challenge orthodoxies of political movements such as fat activism' (Meleo-Erwin 2011: 196).

Blank's arguments are not unusual. In a study of 117 self-identified members of fat/size-acceptance communities, sociologist Carla Pfeffer found that 'only 33 per cent of sample respondents *disagreed* with the statement: "I have engaged in attempts to manage my weight since becoming involved with the fat/size-acceptance community", while 62 per cent *agreed* with the statement: "In the fat/size-acceptance community, some subjects are taboo"' (2012: 19). Furthermore, 'frequently-mentioned taboos included: body projects involving intentional weight management (especially weight-loss surgery and dieting), expressing satisfaction over weight loss, gender and sexual identities and practices, discussions of how fatness may be related to health and/or mobility issues, feelings of dissatisfaction about one's body, and eating disorders' (Pfeffer 2012: 20). Pfeffer's work indicates that 65 per cent of fat activists surveyed both endorse fat/size acceptance and actively attempt to manage their own weight; additionally, 41 per cent of them feel ashamed about these efforts (2012: 21). This recognition of taboos evidences the strife within fat activism over what is allowable discourse; in the face of this strife, it is vital to explore the logics employed by fat activists when confronted with intentional weight loss.

Meleo-Erwin points out that fat activist community responses to Blank's decision to lose weight valorise her efforts as 'life-saving' and acts of 'self-care', appropriating biomedical discourses that 'insist upon fat reduction as urgent matters of risk avoidance and personal health management' (2011: 200). Is there a way around these discourses? Meleo-Erwin says not – there is no outside of the practices that we take up to avoid or reduce obesity-related risks (2011: 201). Certainly, the eagerness with which fat activists marshal health-related claims (albeit more 'positive' ones) to counter mainstream medical discourse demonstrates that even those who want to create more space for fat bodies are heavily invested in (alternative) biomedical discourses. Yet Pfeffer notes 'the potential perils of building liberation-oriented publics around fatness on health-based rather than rights-based ideologies and doctrines' (2012: 30). So I wonder: what about a being in one's body that is not motivated by health fears, by escape from impairment? Can weight loss exemplify a form of fluidity that does not cast aspersions on fatness? I look to the realm of the queer for a clue.

Trans/Fat

In considering the role of fluidity in fat politics and gender/sexual politics, it is tempting to start by reflecting on what seem like obvious parallels between trans people and fat people who intentionally change their body weight.

Seen through the most dominant lens for understanding trans, trans people are understood to intentionally transition from one side of a sex or gender dichotomy to the other on a permanent basis. 'While return may be possible, at its inception the journey is seen as one-way; it is not expected that there will be any turning back' (Ekins and King 2006: 43). Similarly, fat people who intentionally diet or undergo weight loss surgery are typically understood as trying to bring a permanently thinner self into existence (whether or not that is their actual intention).

Transitioning one's sex or gender is frowned upon by a mainstream society heavily invested in the notion of a constant and unchanging dichotomy; the practice has been roundly criticised as well by feminists like Janice Raymond, whose infamous 1979 screed *The Transsexual Empire* argued that transsexualism is a patriarchal practice that medicalises gender identity in order 'to colonize feminist identification, culture, politics and sexuality' (1979: 104). In contrast, transitioning one's body weight from fat to less fat is applauded by a mainstream society heavily invested in preconceived notions of health, beauty and morality; however, the practice has been roundly criticised by fat activists like those in the National Association to Advance Fat Acceptance, which 'condemns gastrointestinal surgery for weight loss under any circumstances' and 'strongly discourages participation in weight-reduction diets' (NAAFA website).

As concerns surgery (for sexual reassignment or weight loss), is there any way to imagine trans people and 'fat losers' as anything but dupes? As anything but tools in a bigger game? By critics, those who intentionally gender-f*ck get read as delusional, trading one extreme for the other, dupes of the gender dichotomy. I'm not sure that fat activism yet has hatched the concept of 'size-f*ck', but let's pretend that it has. Those who intentionally size-f*ck (change their body size, erasing the line between thin and fat) get read as ambitious dieters and sad regainers, dupes of the system. In both cases, observers busy themselves with the ascription of meaning, unconcerned with the self-determination of those whose embodiment they're reading.

One of the most persuasive champions of trans fluidity is Riki Anne Wilchins; from her writing, one does not even need to make a leap to fatness, as she does it herself when she dedicates her work to those who have suffered 'this having one's body and life captured and held hostage, made to bear witness against one's own deepest meanings, this abduction in broad daylight. It is to trans-identified bodies, incested bodies, aging bodies, fat-identified bodies, intersexed bodies, differently abled bodies ... that I write' (Wilchins 1997: 25). Wilchins 'gets' the fat-trans link, using fat often as a parallel: 'The use of bodies to constrain or authorize various meanings and feelings doesn't affect only trans people. Why is it that it is okay in this society to be "fat and lazy", or "fat and jolly", but not "fat and sexy"?' (1997: 131).

Following Foucault, she asks, 'What kind of a system bids us each make of our bodies a problem to be solved, a claim we must defend, or a secret we must publicly confess, again and again?' (Wilchins 1997: 39). Fat activists resist seeing their bodies as problems to be solved, but I think there is more than a touch of the 'fatness as a claim we must defend' perspective in fat community. Wilchins encourages individual self-invention and instability as liberatory tactics, advocating affinity politics: 'Coalitions form around particular issues, and then dissolve. Identity becomes the result of contesting those oppressions, rather than a precondition for involvement. In other words, identity becomes an effect of political activism instead of a cause. It is temporary and fluid, rather than fixed' (Wilchins 1997: 86).

Pfeffer draws a connection between body transition narratives of some trans and fat people, noting that they feel like they're trapped in a body that has become a prison, that they're willing to pursue medical intervention to release their 'true self' (2012: 33). Inasmuch as I reject the logic of a 'true self' that exists outside of performance, perhaps genderqueer or genderfluid, different kinds of narratives that resist essentialism, offer more useful models for thinking about fat bodies that change. Pfeffer asks, 'Do we interpret fat people whose body projects involve medical technologies as tragic, lacking agency, and engaging in a costly and dangerous mutilation of their bodies in a way that is almost a complete inversion of how we might interpret transgender people who choose to use medical technologies such as hormones and surgeries?' (Pfeffer 2012: 35). For fat activists, perhaps the difference lies in the question of permanence. What if it were not the intentional transformation that fat activists rejected, but simply the accompanying notion that the transformation is a lasting one? If fat people who intentionally lose weight say 'I'm doing this now' for whatever the reason – to relieve a perceived burden on the knees, to attempt to resolve diabetes, to fit into certain clothes, to reduce the amount of harassment they attract in public – can it be defensible if they support fat acceptance? Meleo-Erwin suggests so: 'perhaps unlike mainstream individuals, the fat activist grounded in an ethic of body autonomy loses weight from a place of empowerment rather than (solely) from a place of internalised fat-phobia' (2011: 197).

Looking in the mirror, there is something tremendously appealing about Wilchins' embrace of fluidity. A longtime fat studies scholar, I don't have an essential sense of self when it comes to size. I have been an adult for about 24 years now. I have been an average-sized person for about 10 of them, a fat person for about 10 of them, and somewhere in between for the other 4. I do not identify a fat person who has sometimes lost enough weight to be considered average, nor an average person who has sometimes gained so much that I am considered fat. I identify as a change agent. Like a genderqueer person, I like presenting an incoherent identity. I like being fat and not going along with the sense that there's something wrong with being so. I like being average weight and surprising people when I advocate fat pride. I dislike it when fat activism polices its own borders on the basis of who weighs what and how they got to that weight. But I also dislike it when fat activists invest in myths of permanent self-transformation. That is why fluidity is so appealing to me: it offers a model for appreciating where my body is, and how it does politics, as it moves through time and space at different weights. One does not erase the line between thin and fat simply by oscillating between them; that keeps the 'there there'. Like gender transcenders who argue that 'the rigidities of the binary divide constrain us all, and not just those who particularly feel its oppression' (Ekins and King 2006: 183), size transcenders (might I be one of them?) are less interested in passing or assimilation than political activism.

In the *Fat Studies Reader*, Dylan Vade and Sondra Solovay echo Wilchins' perspective:

> We need to recognize that there is no bright line dividing man from woman, fat from thin. Lines just do not work. There are infinite ways to express gender. There are infinitely many different ways to be embodied. No apologies. We must protect the civil rights of everyone, not just those who fit in boxes or fall to extremes on a faulty continuum. If we are going to survive as humans, we need to learn to be with our own difference, to learn to be with the difference around us, to learn from difference, to treasure – and cherish – difference. (2009: 174)

Vade and Solovay's support for infinite forms of expression and embodiment seems to align with Pfeffer's belief that 'taboos against intentional weight loss may be inconsonant with an overall ethics of self-determination and self care' (2012: 24). This perspective leaves the door open for size transcendence. How come we can't imagine changes in weight that don't undermine fat as a reasonable thing to be? Progressives who support genderqueer visions appreciate sexual fluidity, without worrying about whether masculinity or femininity is being undermined in the doing. As appealing as unbridled fluidity is in theory, I am also compelled by those who issue cautions about its overeager embrace.

Caution

Fat activists are not an unreasonable bunch; they recognise that body weight fluctuates – by age, in relation to activity level and food choice. But are they right in saying that efforts at permanent weight loss are really efforts to further malign fatness? Psychologist Deb Burgard, a prominent and passionate advocate for Health at Every Size, notes in a personal interview that attempts by fat people to lose weight, to invest in a permanent transformation, strike her as resonant with reparative therapy, which is marked by efforts to change sexual orientation (always from gay, lesbian or bi to straight, not the other way around). So let's test my theory: Is permanence the sticking point? Not so much for Burgard, who sees the choices we make about eating and movement as fluid practices, separate from identity and body weight. She believes that pursuing weight loss is about wanting to change who you are, whereas pursuing healthy eating and movement is about wanting to change what you do.

Elspeth Probyn offers relevant food for thought in her critique of image-driven identity politics: Fixation on the image, 'translated into identity politics, imparts a hyper surveillance to what bodies look like, and obviates the different feelings bodies experience both in terms of intra-experience (background, personal history, etc.) and inter-experience (in terms of insults, praise, etc.)' (Probyn 2008: 401). It is an interesting point, but Probyn misunderstands the preoccupations of contemporary fat activism, which isn't really obsessed with what bodies look like; rather, it's obsessed with what they *do*, and what their *intentions* are. I contend that fat activists are not fixated on the image, but rather (per Burgard's argument) on performance and rhetoric, which makes an important difference. Moreso than actual body weight, body practices and rhetorics are central to identity and belonging.

Interestingly, Pfeffer contends that 'within fat/size-acceptance publics (which may contain disproportionate numbers of LGBTQ members), there may be greater acceptance of sex and gender-related body transitions than fat and size-related body transitions' (2012: 33). Where do we draw the line? Why is it okay to want to change from M to F or F to M, or to genderf*ck, but it is not okay to want to change from fat to thin, or thin to fat, or to sizef*ck? One answer might lie in the nascence of fat pride as a movement relative to queer social movements. But we also might investigate the perspective of those critics of fluidity who speak from within queer social movements.

For instance, Erin Calhoun Davis's critique of fluidity gives me pause: she claims that queer theoretical valorisations of multiplicity and fluidity 'often overlook or insufficiently recognize the embodied experiences and implications of compulsory gender performance' (2009: 98). In the rush to disrupt stable dichotomies (male/female, fat/thin) with applause for fluidity, we should remember that stable/fluid is itself a false dichotomy, and that fatness is not quite binary in the same way gender has been thought to be. In a time in which 'many young gays and lesbians think of themselves as a part of a "post-gender" world and for them the act of "labelling" becomes a sign of oppression they have happily cast off in order to move into a pluralistic world of infinite diversity' (Halberstam 2005: 19), we see fixed identity rejected in favour of fluid, limitless performance. But in our rush to champion such performance, we may disregard both hegemonic constraints on gender diversity in public interactions, and the disruptive effect of transgressive fluidity not on the gender order, but on individual lives (Davis 2009: 102).

Indeed, critics warn, as appealing as unbridled fluidity seems, there's a hitch. At the same time that transgender bodies have become popular and reliable symbols of fluidity, 'transgenderism also represents a form of rigidity, an insistence on particular forms of recognition, that reminds us of what Martin has called "flexible bodies". Those bodies, indeed, 'that fail to conform to the postmodern fantasy of flexibility that has been projected onto the transgender body may well be punished ... even as they seem to be lauded' (Halberstam 2005: 76–77). Halberstam picks up on Emily Martin's project here, in noting that fantasies of fluidity and flexibility leave most vulnerable those bodies unable or unwilling to change. In a move that is germane to fat activism, Martin seeks to avoid 'the bleakest political consequences of these new models of the ideal flexible body – that, yet again, certain categories of people (women, people of color) will be found wanting. Certain social groups may be seen as having rigid or unresponsive selves and bodies, making them relatively unfit for the kind of society we now seem to desire' (1994: xvii).

Champions of fluidity, take note; we may be riding a wave that drowns the people we most want to protect. It is not helpful to be dominated by a 'liberal individualist notion of subjectivity, in which a postgender subject possesses absolute agency and is able to craft hir gender with perfect felicity' (Salamon 2010: 96). We instead need to consider the power relations that underpin gender structures, and the same goes for fat: be suspicious of any notion of unfettered agency to morph, and examine closely the structures that keep us fat and keep many of us longing to be thin.

Now to return to the point about the nascent state of fat pride that I raised earlier: Perhaps a large part of the problem is that we're not quite 'there' yet. Wilchins writes about trans that 'if we stopped politicising people's bodies and meanings, we'd have more surgery, not less, because changing sex or bodies wouldn't be the socially punishing, economically draining, and psychologically debilitating experience it is now' (1997: 190). Likewise, Peanuts, writing in response to Kirby's blog post castigating fat activists who diet, proclaims:

> Maybe we need a whole new concept. Never mind fat acceptance – what we want to say is EVERY WEIGHT IS OK!!!! So we are in favour of a weight-neutral society!!!! Wouldn't this issue just go away then? If we are in favour of every size, then who cares if someone behind the scenes is changing their body size (or trying to), any more than we'd care about them changing their hairstyle? If everyone is passionately in favour of and working towards people finding it as wonderful as possible to live in whatever body size they happen to be, without pressure to be anything different, and if we are all trying to achieve a

weight-neutral society ... then doesn't that include everyone passionate about size activism? (*Peanuts on The Rotund*, posted 7 September 2007)

I admire the enthusiasm and idealism of both Wilchins and Peanuts, who imagine worlds in which bodies don't quite matter politically the same way they do now. However, politicising people's bodies and meanings is not going to stop any time soon, and the fat body is one of the most highly politicised entities in the panicked fight against 'globesity'.

One way to understand the reticence of fat activists to embrace fluidity at this point in time is to see their investment in what Halberstam has called 'failure as an oppositional tool' (2011: 88). By not dieting, not seeking weight loss surgery, not trying to bring into existence a permanently thinner self, fat failure (partial and inconsistent as it is) refuses to acquiesce to dominant logics of power and discipline (Halberstam 2011: 88). It parallels Lee Edelman's proposition of the queer as 'a relentless form of negativity in place of the forward-looking, reproductive, and heteronormative politics of hope that animates all too many political projects' (Halberstam 2011: 106). Diet culture is forward-looking and hopeful, but perhaps HAES is, too, in as much as it anticipates a time when we stop trying to change who we are.

Future

Marianne Kirby writes, 'If one is actively working to change one's body then one does not accept one's body' (2007). Really? Unless you're my cranky grandmother, you probably don't read many forms of contemporary body modification as evidence of a lack of body acceptance. People pierce, tattoo, apply makeup, colour or cut or grow or shave hair, build muscle, scar, tan, and a hundred other things, and we usually don't read them as deeply mortified about their tattoolessness or on the run from some stigmatised body state. Then again, maybe we do: one school of thought has it that we tan because we're dissatisfied with paleness; we build muscle because we're dissatisfied with flab; we shave because we're embarrassed to be hairy; we put on makeup because we don't like the way our face looks without it. A generation ago, feminists pointed to the myriad ways in which various industries profit off of the insecurity they cultivate in girls and women consumers who will purchase hair colour, eye shadow, tanning sessions, whatever, as a remedy. In the 'post-feminist' moment, we no longer (for the most part) question these practices, merely recognise them as a right, a fun form of self-expression and self-determination.

In the current moment, I would argue that things are different with fatness. Contra the wishes of Peanuts, we haven't reached a place where fat is just another way to be, where fatness has come unmoored from connotations of sickness, immorality and undesirability. Because fat activists must continue to fight the good fight – to find a more neutral or affirmative way to understand fatness – we are (as a whole) still working on 'fat acceptance' that is often (problematically, as I have argued elsewhere) based on the premise of fatness as something that cannot be changed (LeBesco 2004). Those activists who 'understand fat/size acceptance as an ideological commitment to supporting the rights of fat people (no matter one's own size at any given time) rather than a behavioural commitment to not attempting to engage in body projects involving weight management' (Pfeffer 2012: 28) occupy a precarious place in nascent fat politics. My hope for a fat studies that seeks to galvanise fat activism is that we work together on imagining how to advance the movement such that we neither silence nor disappear the diversity of embodied attitudes and practices that currently exists in fat politics – and that we figure out how to give reign to fluidity without demanding it universally.

References

Davis, E.C. 2009. Situating 'fluidity': (Trans) gender identification and the regulation of gender diversity. *GLQ: A Journal of Lesbian and Gay Studies*, 15(1), 97–130.

Ekins, R. and King, D. 2006. *The Transgender Phenomenon*. Thousand Oaks, CA: Sage.

Halberstam, J. 2005. *In a Queer Time and Place: Transgender Bodies, Subcultural Lives*. New York: NYU Press.

Halberstam, J. 2011. *The Queer Art of Failure*. Durham, NC: Duke University Press.

Kirby, M. 2007. Reduced fat. *The Rotund*. [Online] Available at http://www.therotund.com/?p=182 [accessed 1 August 2012].

LeBesco, K. 2004. *Revolting Bodies? The Struggle to Redefine Fat Identity*. Boston: University of Massachusetts Press.

Martin, E. 1994. *Flexible Bodies: Tracking Immunity in American Culture – From the Days of Polio to the Age of AIDS*. Boston: Beacon Press.

Meleo-Erwin, Z. 2011. 'A beautiful show of strength': Weight loss and the fat activist self. *Health* (London), 15(2), 188–205.

Murray, S. 2008. *The 'Fat' Female Body*. New York: Palgrave Macmillan.

Murray, S. 2010. Women under/in control? Embodying eating after gastric banding, in *Whose Weight Is It Anyway? Essays on Ethics and Eating*, edited by S. Vandamme, S. van de Vathorst, and I. de Beaufort. Leuven, Belgium: Acco, 43–54.

National Association to Advance Fat Acceptance. 2012. Official Policies. *National Association to Advance Fat Acceptance*. [Online] Available at http://www.naafaonline.com/dev2/about/docs.html [accessed 7 August 2012].

Nault, C. 2009. 'Punk will never diet': Beth Ditto and the (queer) reevaluation of fat. *Neoamericanist*, 4, 1–14.

Pfeffer, C. 2012. Conflicted alliances: Fatness and competing social publics in the era of the 'obesity epidemic', unpublished manuscript.

Probyn, E. 2008. Silences behind the mantra: Critiquing feminist fat. *Feminism and Psychology*, 18, 401–4.

Raymond, J.G. [1979] 1994. *The Transsexual Empire: The Making of the She-Male*. New York: Teachers College Press.

Salamon, G. 2010. *Assuming a Body: Transgender and Rhetorics of Materiality*. New York: Columbia University Press.

Vade, D. and Solovay, S. 2009. No apology: Shared struggles in fat and transgender law, in *The Fat Studies Reader*, edited by E. Rothblum and S. Solovay. New York: New York University Press, 167–175.

Wilchins, R.A. 1997. *Read My Lips: Sexual Subversion and the End of Gender*. Milford, CT: Firebrand.

Chapter 6
Chubby Boys with Strap-Ons: Queering Fat Transmasculine Embodiment

James Burford and Sam Orchard

Introduction

Rooster Tails is a weekly web-comic that has followed Sam Orchard's transition from 'shy girl' to 'awkward semi-butch chubby nerd' since 2010. Orchard's comic has contributed to an emerging archive of cultural work around fat transgender embodiment, including among others, Wyatt Riot's writing and video work and the writing and tumblring of Mey DJneres (e.g. 2013). Our present text is nourished by an emerging community of scholarship that connects transgender embodiment, food and body size (see Bergman 2009, Cooper 2012, Watson-Russel 2012). In activist conversations, and increasingly in academic ones (e.g. Vade and Solovay 2009), the connections between transgender and fat rights struggles have been articulated. A clear pathway into analysis has been to examine the ways in which both fat and trans* people, and fat trans* people, are expected to reproduce societal value systems – that is: fat people *should* want to become thin, and trans* people *should* want to be model examples of the binary gender system. Often, these values emerge through the figures of the 'trans* person trapped in the wrong body' and/or 'thin person trapped in a fat body'. Orchard's comics trouble both of these accounts, and therefore have the potential to prompt and invigorate future conversations in the intersecting fields of trans* and fat studies. While not intended as such, we also suggest our work might serve as a response to some fat studies research, and conversations in fat activisms, that make encompassing claims about representing trans* fat embodiment by invoking acronyms like LGBT. Too often we have found that such promises of inclusion fail to deliver. Indeed, sometimes the 't' appears to be mere relish adorning and 'inclusifying' the main meal of lesbian and gay studies. This is an issue we address, in a small way, by publishing a conversation between two people who (at the time of writing) shelter under the broad trans* umbrella, and focus on accounts of fat embodiment in trans* cultural work.

Our text is a co-constructed conversation between the two authors. It is a product of an extended series of email exchanges during the early months of 2013, which were then worked into a dialogic text. In taking up this methodology of representation, we intended to create a 'messy text' (Marcus 1998) – a break with the representational technologies of traditional writing forms. We are attracted to the potential of such texts to resist dichotomous thinking by proliferating different and indeed divergent accounts. Working in this way frees us as authors to disagree with each other, and ourselves. In response, we invite you (the reader) to read this text differently. Obviously, the images we have included are an important part of the work of this text. As for the conversation itself, we suggest you might wish to read it aloud. Perhaps you will notice which senses are activated, what thoughts come to mind, and which feelings are evoked. Consider which of our words you may wish to spit out, and those you wish to savour. We'd ask you, too, to observe the moments where you might wish to speak back – what is it that you want to say, and how do you want to say it?

Sam, it's a real pleasure to have a chance to speak to you about your comics. I'd like to begin by acknowledging that yours is an autobiographical project about your transition, so your body and the changes it goes through are always in your comics, and will be at the centre of our talk. It is then – in a spirit of co-authorial fairness – that I'd also like to 'come out' about my embodiment. Rather than tell (my? a?) story its traditional way from 'the beginning', I'd like to start with right now. From the perspective of an outsider looking at me as I type, I imagine (fantasise) they would see me as a camp, cis-male person who is plump. If they were to address me, they would almost certainly use male pronouns. If they looked harder still they might notice my queer deportment, my large rings, my too-sweet fragrance, and colourful clothing. My size would likely go unremarked, except perhaps as tall, or 'solid'. When I chat with my doctor, they sometimes admonish me to lose some weight, but are generally surprised to find out that, according to abstract measures such as the BMI, my body falls within the 'obese' category (maybe I've been training?). Unfortunately, this 'coming out' doesn't really satisfy me. It doesn't tell much about my own attachments, the way my body has travelled through time, or my subjective feelings about it – and perhaps such a story is for another chapter. I would like the reader to be in possession of a couple of extra clues however. While today I may be read as both relatively 'male' and 'average' sized, my body bears the marks of weight loss, and gain. I am also a person who has lived experience of non-normative gender identity and expression, and the social costs and many pleasures associated with this.

Sam, in looking through Rooster Tails *from 2010 to the present it's clear that over the years there have been some changes in the way you draw yourself. You seem to have become bigger in the comic, and increasingly represent yourself with a squishy tummy. Does this represent changes to your own body over this time, or is it more about your increasing comfort around including the fullness of your body in your work?*

I think the changes are a combination of my drawing ability/style, actual changes in my body size, and my increasing comfort with my own fatness. When I first started *Rooster Tails*, I drew all characters with big heads and skinny necks/ bodies. This was probably a result of my drawing ability and finding my own style, as well as my level of comfort with fatness in general.

I think that my consciousness of fat-phobia and fat-pride has been developing over the last four years, and that gets reflected through the increasingly diverse body shapes I draw in my comics. My critical consciousness around fat issues is in constant development, and has also been very much connected to my transition (by transition I don't mean medical interventions of testosterone – although that has played a part in changing my body shape – I mean thinking about and embodying ways of living as a transmasculine person).

As a young girl I was very conscious of weight. I was a chubby teen, and felt very uncomfortable about my tummy. I spent a good number of years with my arms wrapped around my waist, in an attempt to hide my stomach. For teenage women weight is seen as an indicator of attractiveness, and certainly my weight contributed to my feeling that I was 'failing' at being a girl. When I came out as someone who was attracted to women, and entered into dyke communities, I was surprised and heartened by the level of acceptance around body diversity, and how my chubbiness contributed to making me a 'successful' butch. Then, as I began transitioning towards the masculine/boy end of the gender spectrum, and engaging with gay male and transmale communities, I began experiencing body-policing again. This was obviously different to that which I experienced as a girl, but involved similar messages around 'fat is bad/unattractive'. Within small gay male communities, I felt as though I had to be super skinny, or super ripped to be attractive to other men. Within transmasculine communities, I felt as though weight was seen as feminine, or, rather, as feminising, as in: 'urgh, look at my curves'. Then, as I moved to larger queer communities, with more bear scenes, the discourses around 'sexiness' and body weight changed again.

These transitions and differing community expectations caused me to think about weight and body issues. As well as the fact that I have a partner who finds chubby people attractive. It has caused me to examine my relationship with my body, as well as my relationship to different communities' values around body weight and attractiveness. I think over time I've made a point of talking about chubby bodies, particularly chubby trans* bodies, in a positive way, so as to disrupt some of those negative discourses. And, as I am a chubby transguy myself, who writes an autobiographical comic, depicting my own embodiment has been a part of that.

As a reader, I appreciate the intimacy of your work, in particular your willingness to allow us to witness paradoxical thoughts. I'm thinking here of a series of comics in 2011 which explored your feelings about your own body size. You indicated that you were planning to lose *weight in order to feel more comfortable binding in the heat and humidity of Auckland, but also because your endocrinologist told you to (see Figure 6.1). These accounts sit alongside others in your collection which are more assertive, calling out fat phobia, and proliferating positive images of chubby trans* guys. In bringing this up, it's not my intention to point out 'bad (fat) politics', instead I am interested in how these kinds of inconsistencies are actually quite consistent with my own experience, and possibly the experiences of others who are not thin. Even though, as a queer and feminist knowledge worker, I critique discourses around body normativities, I do at times, actually quite often, desire to be thinner. I also, with varying degrees of commitment, engage in exercise. Increasingly, this is exercise that I frame as a project around feeling good about moving in my body, but other times, if I am honest, it is undertaken by a disciplining self who wants to trim and tighten. Being able to see these moments of ambivalence in your work is important for me as a reader. It is an invitation to reflect on the messiness of practicing a progressive fat politics, and experiencing our own desires about our bodies in a world structured by fat-shaming and obesity hysteria. How do you feel about these paradoxes in your work?*

Like you said, these inconsistencies have been consistent with how I experience, and value, my body. Just as we live in a heterosexist/cissexist world and we have to constantly deal with our own internalised homo/trans phobias, so too do we have to deal with our internalised fat phobias in a fat phobic world.

For me, I have found it really hard to work out how to love myself, and love my body, in the face of a world that quite consistently points out its unattractiveness. Whether I'm unattractive because I'm a perceived-female-bodied butch person, a perceived-male-bodied femme person (or just a generally non-normatively gendered person), or I'm unattractive because I'm queer-looking, or I'm unattractive 'cause I have curves, it all impacts my self-esteem. It also makes it hard to fight against, in a world where mass media bombards me with messages that whatever I'm doing with my body, I'm 'not doing it right'. So, yeah, I think my analysis is fraught, 'cause *I* feel fraught about it. *I* find it hard to keep positive, and to continue loving myself when the world is telling me I shouldn't.

I don't see people like me on television or in films, I've never seen someone who looks like me being portrayed as attractive. I feel really sad about that. I feel sad because I can't change mainstream media. I feel sad that I buy into it. I feel sad that even when my boyfriend tells me that he finds me/my body attractive, I think he's only saying that to be 'nice' to me. On a political level, I know that fat phobia exists, and it's awful, and I can be critical of it – but I also feel the impacts of it, and know it influences how I feel about myself, and that's incredibly disheartening. I want to be able to be empowered and stand up and say 'fuck you all, my body is fearless, and amazing, and curvy and delicious!' and sometimes I can, and I do that. So, I think that the inconsistencies in my comics are a reflection of where I'm at.

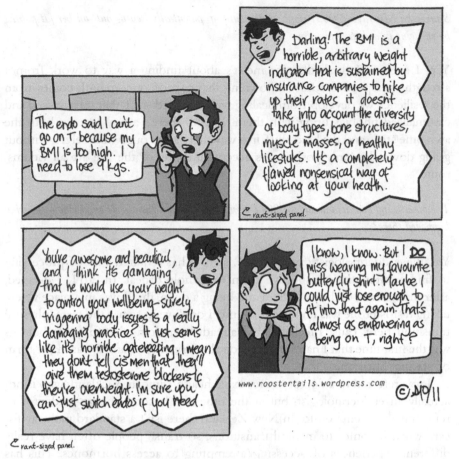

Figure 6.1 Trying to find the silver lining
Source: Courtesy of Rooster Tails Comics.

Yes, I think this is an important issue to talk about in a number of activist communities, where there seems to be an expectation that our politics will neatly fit with our experience. That we won't, or at least shouldn't feel ashamed, guilty or depressed about our bodies, and if we do this should be quickly tidied up and repackaged. Reflecting back on my community development practice, I am aware that I have done this myself. I recall facilitating a support group and trying to steer conversations about fatness away from painful, complex or ambivalent feelings and toward 'good' ones, like pride. But I feel we can lose something when we do this, potentially something quite critical. This phenomenon of paradoxes seems to connect with some important articles I have read in the field of fat studies, like Robyn Longhurt's (2011) autoethnography about her experience of simultaneously critiquing and desiring slimness, and Karen Throsby and Debra Gimilin's (2010) work in the same vein. It also reminds me of

Samantha Murray's (2005) work on the guilt of potentially 'selling out' on her fat politics by engaging in a dieting practice.

Yep, I agree – I think that for me it's about finding a way to work from a strengths perspective, while still owning that part of our strength comes from the resilience we develop from dealing with the hard stuff that internalised and externalised phobias bring with them. I think there's a way to own both the awesome stuff and the hard stuff in a way that values our whole selves, without going down the 'only positivity is accepted' route, or the 'we are all victims' route.

The other thing I noticed about the 2011 comic was the line about your endocrinologist, what happened there?

Yes, the endocrinologist experience … sigh. It has required a lot of processing to find a 'strengths' perspective from the whole ordeal. In 2011, I decided, after many years, of living as Sam and being a dude, that I was in a place where taking testosterone was important for me. I don't want to use the term 'physical transition' here, 'cause I feel like I had already been doing that for years, but this was the first time that I had sought medical interventions, and it was in the form of starting hormones.

I was referred to a doctor at the sexual health clinic in Auckland, who is not actually an endocrinologist, but at the time had become the go-to doctor to refer trans* patients on to. In New Zealand there isn't a standard pathway for care when it comes to medical transitions, so trans* people often have really different experiences of accessing/attempting to access hormones. This has been outlined in the New Zealand Human Rights Commission's report *To be who I am/Kia noho au ki toku ano ao*, which has found that the provision of public health services to be 'patchy and inconsistent [with] major gaps in availability, accessibility, acceptability and quality of medical services required by a trans* person seeking to transition' (2008: 50). In this instance, the doctor in question had set criteria that he used to assess whether he would write prescriptions for hormones. One criterion that he used was weight. He used the BMI to assess me, and said he would only prescribe me testosterone if I lost 9kgs.

I felt like I'd been kicked in the guts. The whole process left me feeling heartbroken and humiliated. I had been living as a guy for three years at that point, had been thinking about gender my whole life, and had finally decided that I felt 'ready' to begin taking testosterone. Instead of an informed consent model, where a doctor points out the risks and benefits of medical intervention (which I had already researched myself when it came to testosterone), I felt like I was being told by a father figure 'no, you're not allowed that, you haven't been good enough, show me that you really want it and then maybe I'll let you'.

This was a first for me. No doctor had ever told me to lose weight, or refused to prescribe me medication because of my weight. I went home and researched the BMI, and found out about how problematic it is around gender (as well as culture/race). I had no idea whether my doctor was using the scale for me as a 'female' or 'male', he never explained to me why the BMI was important in terms of transitioning, he just told me that I should lose the weight or it would be too 'dangerous' to prescribe me testosterone, and that I should probably join Weight Watchers or Jenny Craig (I was a student at the time, with no disposable income, which meant this was a financial impossibility from the outset).

I talked to my partner, and to close friends (I was too humiliated at the time to talk with others about it), and got reassurance that he was a dick … but I still took the doctor's words on board. Doctors were supposed to know best, they were supposed to be kind, they were supposed to know how to keep us healthy – was I being precocious thinking that I knew better than him? Was I making excuses about my body? I felt like a failure. And I felt angry at myself for feeling like a failure. As I look back on it now, this comic reminds me of that feeling of holding that inconsistent subjectivity – simultaneously feeling outraged as well as awful and insecure. I wanted to punch the doctor, but I also felt that I really had to lose the weight because otherwise I would continue to be a 'bad fat person' who didn't 'deserve' to go on T.[1] It was really rough. In my comics I often use Joe (the character of my boyfriend) as a sounding board to explore alternative perspectives on an issue. This was true for one of my comics around this issue (Figure 6.1); I felt like I was oscillating between Joe's outrage and my own shame.

I recall that time myself, both reading your comic and talking with you. I remember feeling angry about the way you had been treated, and a kind of aching despair that trans* friends, and some of the university students I was doing advocacy with, seemed compelled to follow often mindless medical dictates, not only with regard to fatness, but around gender identity too. But in this case you kind of outmanoeuvred the doctor, right? Joe organised a fundraiser among friends so you could pay to go to another endo' who gave you the prescription.

Yes, in the end I knew that I would end up in a much worse position (physically and emotionally) if I tried to lose the weight. It would impact my self-esteem, my relationship with my body (which was already quite fraught), my relationship to food (which is a huge part of my self-care), and my relationship with Joe. It also felt like I was colluding with the doctor, and I really didn't feel like I could do that. So, yeah, I was lucky enough to have a partner who fundraised for me to go to a private endocrinologist, and bypass the public system altogether. It meant that I didn't battle to change the structural oppression, but it did enable

---

1 Testosterone.

me to get the interventions I needed. It's important to acknowledge here that not everyone has the resources, whether financial or cultural, to beat the system in this way.

For the next couple of questions, I'd like to broaden out our conversation to examine the social context in which your work is produced. It is clear that discussions about fat are not only common with health workers. As you touched on earlier, discussions about fatness seem to take particular routes in transmasculine communities and media. How have you seen these play out?

There's some real diversity in the way that weight is discussed in various communities, a majority of the time there is a 'fat = bad' message, but that can come from a variety of places. Part of identity is about finding yourself in the reflection of others. I had never seen a transmasculine person (that I knew of) on television or in real life before I was 24. The only one I can think of was Hilary Swank's Brandon Teena in *Boy's Don't Cry*, and I had always seen that character written about as a lesbian who dressed like a boy, so I didn't make the 'trans' connection. I had no idea that we existed. So, when I met my first transguy and things clicked into place ('aha! that is me too!'), I began looking for more and more reflections. I was living in Dunedin, a small city in the South Island, so there was a tiny pool of transguys to pester.

I took to the Internet, as I had when coming out as someone who liked women, to see what I could find. My experiences of Internet-based transmasculinity, through tumblrs, Facebook groups, etc., were often white-centric and skinny. These groups told me that curves were bad – because 'girls' had curves, and so being less feminine meant being skinny, or being muscly, but definitely not being curvy. This seemed particularly true for noho (no masculinising hormones) boys (like me at the time) – without testosterone redistributing fat away from your hips and butt, you should do everything in your power to make them as small as possible, because that would mean you would be more likely to 'pass'. Passing is a fraught term, and is not the ideal for everyone, but that is a whole other discussion.

I have noticed a couple of alternative discourses that constitute fat transmasculine embodiment in seemingly contradictory ways. My primary exposure is to a discourse which emphasises the benefits of losing fat, or more specifically engaging in diet and exercise in order to try and lose certain curves that might normatively be read as cis-feminine, in favour of 'angularity'. An example of this can be seen in a post by blogger Elliot DeLine on the website originalplumming. com. He observed that his ideal transmasculine embodiment would be 'the cute, skinny, hipster boy' or the 'intellectual, emo twink' (DeLine 2012). We can also see this in the work of Kyle Lukoff who speaks about his experience with anorexia, and his attempts to 'starv[e] away' breasts and hips (Lukoff 2010: 123). But DeLine's skinny, hipster boy seems quite a different kind of transmasculine embodiment to that described by S. Bear Bergman in hir chapter 'Part-time Fatso' (2009). In this work Bergman positions 'bulk' as something that can be helpful for giving male cues.

I think there are some interesting differences between the 'socially acceptable weight' in different community contexts. There's something about bulk that can be read as a masculine indicator. This is true for when I'm being read in the context of bear communities; not being a twink is regarded hot. Similarly, in heterosexual cis-male spaces, size can be read as relating to power, and being able to take up space. It's interesting that fatness, thinness and muscle bulk can be seen as positives for male/masculine people, whereas women/feminine people are supposed to be neither muscular nor fat. I feel as though there's a bit more room to move within male spaces.

I feel that when I'm being read as a woman, or within transmasculine communities, my weight is more likely to be seen as a sign of weakness. It is more likely to be read within discourses around failure – too curvy to be seen as male, or too fat to be attractive. The weakness is expressed through the related ideas that fatness is a result of 'not having enough self-control/discipline', or being 'too lazy'.

Bergman has also reflected on the significant differences ze has encountered in public space whether ze is read as a fat woman or transmasculine butch person, as ze puts it ze is 'Fat one minute (as a woman) and just a big boy in the next', with resulting differences in whether ze is assumed to want a diet coke or a side of fries. Mey DJneres (2013) has also examined this from her perspective as a fat trans woman, noting that when she began presenting as a woman her size became 'fair play' for both public negativity as well as fetishisation. Have you noticed changes in the way your body is received as you have transitioned?

I was more likely to be policed around my body when I presented as a girl. It seems more socially acceptable to offer suggestions, or just plain make assumptions about food choices (like that you should be drinking diet coke if you're a woman, or that you shouldn't be ordering the extra-large with a side of whatever). I have definitely noticed a shift in the portion sizes that I'm given in dining halls, or even at friend's places – I'll be offered more, and seconds, without hesitation these days. Whereas before, people seemed to be embarrassed (I was definitely also embarrassed) to offer me seconds, thirds, or fourths – because it is seen as 'breaking the rules' or shameful for girls to eat a lot. When I was younger, my brothers and I would have eating competitions at home. But, as I became a teenager, it became 'gross', 'unladylike' and embarrassing for everyone if I tried to partake in those sorts of competitions.

Chubby Boys with Strap-Ons

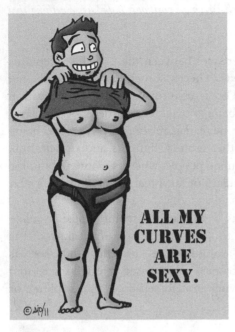

Figure 6.2   All my curves

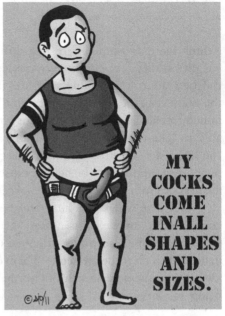

Figure 6.3   All shapes

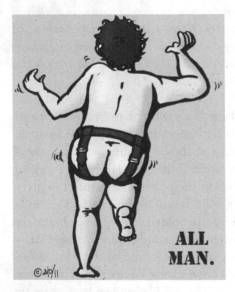

Figure 6.4   All man

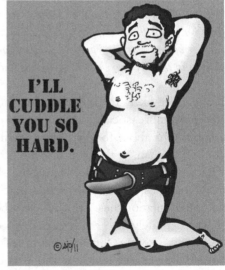

Figure 6.5   Cuddle you

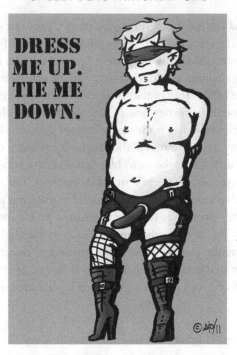

Figure 6.6   Dress up

Source: All figures courtesy of Rooster Tails Comics.

Now I'd like to talk about your 2011 collection 'Chubby boys with strap-ons' (see figures 6.2–6.6). As we have spoken about previously, fatness, or as you have put it 'curviness' is often constituted as feminine, or pre-transition. In particular, the curves of the chest, butt and thighs, which are often read as indexing cis-feminine embodiment. Was 'Chubby boys with strap-ons' a direct response to this?

Yes! I wanted to create art that would disrupt the audience(s).

I wanted to have a direct conversation with the transmasculine Internet communities that I had engaged with to disrupt the value that was being placed on skinny (white) transmasculine bodies. I wanted to show that boys with curves are hot, boys of all colours are hot. It was intended to be a 'fuck you, I'm sexy' response to the common discourses that I felt de-valued me.

The other direct conversation I wanted to have was with a cis-centric audience. I had drawn an illustration of Wolverine a few years ago for my university magazine's queer issue. The picture was of Wolverine wearing just boots and a harness with a bright yellow dildo. It was really wonderful how many cis-centric people just didn't understand it – 'why is he wearing a strap-on if he's a guy?' I wanted to recreate this image with more 'real' transboys (because as much as I'd like Wolverine to be trans*, I am not sure that any of the X-Men creators really envisioned that for him). The idea of having erotic boys wearing strap-ons with dildos, in empowered poses, felt like it was an important disruption of what sexiness could look like, and what sexy men could look like.

I think that one of the things that happens when we live in a phallo-centric society is that the penis becomes one of the most central thoughts for people. This seems especially true for both sexuality and gender identity; with cis gay men it seems society gets fascinated about which partner's dick goes into what orifice, with cis lesbians there seems to be a focus on questioning about whether you can 'really' have sex if there's no dick present, with trans women the conversations revolve around whether she still has got 'that part' or if she's 'had the surgery', and the opposite is true for transguys. So I wanted to really disrupt that conversation – to show a silicone phallus – to highlight the construction of gender (they literally put on their dicks, or dildos, depending on how they identify) – to show that a silicone dick/dildo is just as sexy as one made from skin and nerves – to disrupt the idea that trans bodies are somehow 'lacking' or 'embarrassing'.

'All my curves are sexy' (Figure 6.2) and 'All man' (Figure 6.4) seem like important pieces of work. In the first of these you have created a transmasculine figure with a large and unbound chest, and in the second a figure with large hips and butt. But it is not only the images that do work. Throughout this collection the text also seems to assert different modes of discourse about the transmasculine body. What I find most striking is the way that it creates an erotic politics for fat trans guys. Your boys are naked and erect. They look directly at us and smile, or dance. It seems they are not only celebrated – but you have gone further and positioned curvy-transmasculine embodiment as both desired and desirable. Your boys are sexy, and they know it.

Yes they are! I think a lot of the time I have felt that I (and people with my body type/shape/gender identity) should feel ashamed, ugly and undesirable. So this was a reaction to that. These boys love the way they look. I especially love the 'All my curves are sexy' boy (Figure 6.2), because he is being cheeky, and proudly showing off his curvy chest. I think that's so important, especially since a really dominant narrative around trans* people is that we hate our bodies, and transguys especially hate the parts that are seen to be 'feminine' like our hips and our breasts/chests/pecs.

Your project seems fabulously queer. Not only does your work queer transmasculine embodiment and identity, by proliferating alternative and (to some) incoherent images and accounts of masculinities, it seems to me that your comic makes an important contribution to queering fat transmasculine embodiment by your representation of yourself, and your boys, as masculine and chubby, desirable and desired. Can we expect more work of this kind?

I hope that my work will continue to challenge norms of desire, and celebrate difference. Part of the reason I started creating comics was because there was a lack of media that represented and celebrated me and the people that I love. I spent a long time feeling sad about that, and critiquing it, and then felt empowered enough to say 'fuck it, if "they're" not going to create it, then I am'. I have so many questions and I love complications in our embodiments and our identities – I find that interesting and compelling, so I think that I'll just keep exploring that stuff, asking questions, trying things, and see what happens.

References

Bergman, S.B. 2009. Part-time fatso, in *The Fat Studies Reader*, edited by S. Solovay and E. Rothblum. New York: New York University Press, 139–142.

Cooper, C. 2012. A queer and trans fat activist timeline: Queering fat activist nationality and cultural imperialism. *Fat Studies: An Interdisciplinary Journal of Body Weight and Society*, 1(1), 61–74.

DeLine, E. 2012. Timid boy, eating. *Original Plumming*. [Online, 9 February] Available at: http://www.originalplumbing.com/2012/02/09/timid-boy-eating/ [accessed 3 May 2013].

DJneres, M. 2013. Fat, trans and (working on being) fine with it. *Autostraddle*. [Online, 28 March] Available at: http://www.autostraddle.com/fat-trans-and-working-on-being-fine-with-it-168108/ [accessed 3 May 2013].

Human Rights Commission. 2007. To be who I am/kia noho au ki toku ano ao, the report of the Transgender Inquiry, Human Rights Commission.

Longhurst, R. 2011. Becoming smaller: Autobiographical spaces of weight loss *Antipode*, 44(3), 1–21.

Lukoff, K. 2010. Taking up space, in *Gender Outlaws: The Next Generation*, edited by K. Bornstein and S.B. Bergman, Berkeley: Seal Press, 122–127.

Marcus, G. 1998. *Ethnography through Thick and Thin*. Princeton: Princeton University Press.

Murray, S. 2005. Doing politics or selling out? Living the fat body. *Women's Studies: An Inter-disciplinary Journal*, 34(3–4), 265–277.

Throsby, K. and Gimilin, D. 2010. Critiquing thinness and wanting to be thin, in *Secrecy and Silence in the Research Process: Feminist Reflections*, edited by R. Ryan-Flood and R. Gill, Oxon Routledge, 105–116.

Vade, D. and Solovay, S. 2009. No apology: Shared struggles in fat and transgender law, in *The Fat Studies Reader*, edited by E. Rothblum and S. Solovay, New York: New York University Press, 167–175.

Watson-Russel, D. (2012). *Growing Boys: Trans* Male Narratives on Food and the Construction of Bodies*, unpublished dissertation, La Trobe University.

Chapter 7
Causing a Commotion: Queering Fat in Cyberspace

Cat Pausé

Queer *(a)*: Deviating from the expected or normal.

To queer *(v)*: To ruin or thwart.[1]

The World Wide Web has introduced possibilities for the engagement of fat activism. This chapter explores how fat activists engage in queering fat online. It considers five examples of the ways fatness has been queered within cyberspace and ruminates on whether queering fat online is a useful tool in fat politics.

Queer Theory

Queer is often understood as an umbrella term; a word which encapsulates a differentiation from the heteronormative discourse (see Jagose 1996 for an exploration of the term queer and its various usage). Heteronormative discourse is discourse that reinforces existing power structures and understandings of individuals drawn from essentialist assumptions. Queer theory, in its use by academics and activists alike, allows for a method to disrupt (and deconstruct) dominant assumptions and challenge the privilege of dominant groups. Butler (1993) suggests that queering allows for the creation of discomfort and the making of noise. While queer theory, and the use of queering, began within the realm of questioning the essential nature of gender and sexual orientation, its use has grown to encapsulate a larger area of critical studies which examine race, ethnicity, ability, class, and body size. In challenging the positions of essential, normal, and natural, queering is (or can be) a useful tool in the examination of fatness and the lived experience of body diversity within culture.

Queering has been used in a range of academic disciplines, including early childhood education (Janmohamend 2010, Robinson 2005, Sears 1999), geography (Gibson-Graham 1999), public administration (Lee, Learmonth and Harding 2008), Asian studies (Rofel 2012), and religious studies (LePeau 2007).

---

1 The free dictionary, online.

Some scholars use queering as a way to challenge essentialist positions; others use queering as a framework for subverting existing epistemologies. In similar ways, queering may be used by fat studies scholars and fat activists alike to disrupt the normative beliefs and acceptable standards around body size.

Queering Fat

Fat activists have engaged in such queering across the globe, organising fat synchronised swimming groups, fat burlesque troupes, and the Fattylympics (Cooper and Murray 2012). By challenging beliefs around fatness, these activities queer fatness. By providing an opportunity for fat women to wear lingerie and dance in provocative manners for others to watch, fatness is queered by fat burlesque troops. In organising fat women to train and perform as synchronised swimmers, groups such as Aquarporko queer fatness (*Aquaporko! The Documentary* 2013). While they may wear pink flowered swim caps, these fat swimming ladies do not look like Esther Williams. These in-person activities allow for fat individuals to make noise and cause discomfort; they also allow for participants to engage in a celebration of their fat bodies and the fat lives that they lead. These activities, however, are usually limited to the individuals who create them, or those who reside in the areas where such opportunities exist. By taking some activities online, spaces are opened up to individuals around the world who are able to participate through the use of the World Wide Web.

The Internet

On the Internet, many groups have found a place to create safe spaces for their members. The Internet allows individuals from minority groups to present an opposing picture of their identity, pushing back against the normative discourse. One such space is the fat-o-sphere, a subculture of fat people online that promotes fat positivity (Harding and Kirby 2009). For many in the fat community,[2] participation in the fat-o-sphere allows opportunities for kinship, self-expression, and being heard (Pausé 2012). Fat people write blogs, maintain Tumblrs, and share tips and tricks for living the fat life through a variety of channels. The fat-o-sphere, in this context, is a hub of oppositional fat politics (Kahn and Kellner 2004).

The Internet also allows for the exposure of the fat community to the rest of the world. Someone may stumble upon the fat-o-sphere, and be introduced to ideas and perspectives they have never considered. Others may actively seek

---

2 See Introduction by Wykes for background on the fat activist community.

out this space of positivity, seeking a different discourse of fatness. Unlike the mainstream media representations of fatness (concerning globesity and negative fat tropes), representations in the fat-o-sphere are vast and variable. Rather than the familiar fat trope (the unhealthy, unhappy, miserable fat person who wishes desperately to find and free the thin person inside), a diverse representation of fat identities, fat embodiment, and fat lives are showcased around the fat-o-sphere.

The five examples selected demonstrate a range of activities that queer fatness in cyberspace. They are by no means an exhaustive exploration of the various campaigns, representations, and endeavours that exist throughout the fat-o-sphere; these five were selected because they showcase a range of the kinds of activities afforded by the functionalities of the Internet and because they are well known in the online fat community.

The Campaign

The *I Stand* campaign was begun by Marilyn Wann, a well-known fat activist in the San Francisco Bay area and the author of *Fat!So?* (Wann 2012). It was created as a response to a fat shaming campaign that targeted children in the state of Georgia, USA. The Georgia campaign, *Strong4Life*, featured ads of fat children and the phrase 'WARNING' in red lettering across the bottom, along with a statement about childhood obesity (e.g., 'It's hard to be a little girl when you're not'). The purpose of the ads, according to the campaign, was to bring attention to childhood obesity and encourage parents to take the issue seriously. Concerns about the negative tone and shaming nature of the ads, however, were raised by those in the public health sector, the eating disorders community, and fat activists alike (Lohr 2012).

Wann's response, the *I Stand* campaign, took direct aim at the image and message of the ads themselves. Wann invited individuals to submit a photo of themselves and their position (a statement about what they 'stand for' in relation to weight/stigma/health), which were then made into a poster for the I Stand campaign. Each poster has a picture of an individual and a statement about what they stand for. The phrase 'I STAND' is found in bright pink lettering across the bottom, along with fat positive statement. The first poster, featuring Marilyn Wann, read 'I STAND against harming fat children. Hate/= health'.

Most of the submissions came from fat individuals, but a range of body sizes can be found among the collection. The posters may be found on the 'I Stand Against Weight Bullying' Tumblr (Wann 2012).

Contributions range from 'I STAND for body diversity', 'I STAND against teaching kids to hate their bodies', 'I STAND for doing what you love in front of those who doubt you', 'I STAND for taking up space', and 'I STAND for

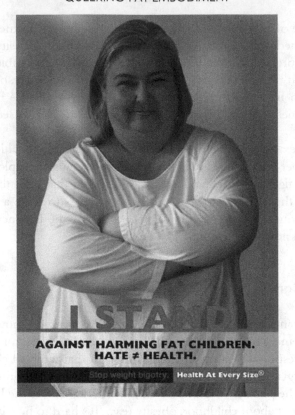

Figure 7.1 I Stand
Source: Courtesy of Marilyn Wann.

doing what you love in the body you have now' (Wann 2012). Each poster ends with, 'Stop weight bigotry. Health at Every Size'.

Wann's I Stand campaign allows for individuals of all sizes to present positive messages about fatness, body size, and physical health and well-being. Using the same format as posters intended to fat-shame children, but changing the message to fat positivity, queers fat. By allowing others to produce the pictures and text, I Stand fosters user created content within a larger campaign for social change. The campaign, however, was not without critics.

As noted in an open letter from the people of caucus of NOLOSE,[3] 'A response to white fat activism from People of Color in the fat justice movement', too many fat activist projects represent only a singular point of view (Shuai et al. 2012). Shuai et al. cautioned against allowing the fat justice movement to

---

3 'NOLOSE is a volunteer-run organization dedicated to ending the oppression of fat people and creating vibrant fat queer culture' (NOLOSE).

become separated along class and colour lines, and they noted that the power of social media allows for connections to be made, conversations to be had, and for a diverse group of individuals to engage in the planning, execution, and promotion of any work being done.

Within the letter, the authors present many ways that those who engage in fat activism may work towards being inclusive. Being aware of differing kinds of privilege is one, as well is reflecting on an individual's own privilege and actions which reinforce oppression against others. Being mindful of the impact the work may have on those from other racial, ethnic, and class backgrounds. Another step would be to not fall into the trap of asking others, outside of our own groups, to educate us about the issues of oppression faced by them. Most importantly, those who claim commitment to these issues must assume responsibility for ensuring that a range of voices are included.[4] As noted in the letter from NOLOSE:

> Sending out an invitation for all contacts to participate is not the same as doing the thoughtful work of being inclusive, which requires planning, communication among groups, and transparency. Blanket invitation through social media, or "crowd sourcing", returns a large response from those already closely related to the issue, who often share the initiator's stance, privileges, and power. (Shuai et al. 2012)

The Activist

Kath Read is an Australian fat activist who has a large presence in the fat-o-sphere. Found on her blog The Fat Heffalump (and related Tumblr, Facebook, Instagram, and Twitter platforms), Kath writes about her own experiences as a fat woman living in a less than friendly environment (Read 2013a). The tagline for The Fat Heffalump is 'Living with Fattitude', and Kath invites others to be observers to her doing just that.

Kath writes about her fat identity, her fat embodiment, her fat fashion, and her fat life. She shares stories of triumph, and stories of harassment. She posts pictures of herself in her outfit of the day (otherwise known in cyberspace as OOTD), and often addresses the fat hate and fat shame she observes in the mainstream media, news, and her everyday life.

Occasionally Kath will write a piece like 'You're not the first person to tell a fat person', in which she addresses common myths about fatness, and provides answers to some comments that she frequently receives when she has

---

4 It should be noted that this text has failed to ensure a representation of diverse voices across fat activism and fat studies.

an influx of new readers (Read 2013b). In these posts, Kath is providing the opportunity for those who are reading to educate themselves a bit more about the assumptions they hold and beliefs they forget to unpack. She assumes the role of a teacher, answering the questions of her students in thoughtful and reflective ways.

Kath also speaks to her frustration about having to always educate the ignorant; it isn't her job, she tells the readers, to highlight their bigotry, suggest they do their homework, or point out when they are being oppressive.

Simply through living her life online, Kath Read queers what it is to be fat. Her lack of shame, her love of fashion, and her brightly coloured hair, all contradict what fatness is supposed to be. She may invite others to join her, but it is the testimony of her life she is sharing with the web. She refuses to live her life according to other people's standards, and she has long since forgotten that she is supposed to wait to live her dreams until she's achieved the state of thinness.

The ECourse

Individuals interested in embarking on their own journey to fat positivity are able to participate in an online course, hosted by Rachele at *The Nearsighted Owl*, called 'How to be a fat bitch ECourse' (Cateyes 2013a). The ECourse runs for 52 weeks and began in early 2013, although users are welcome to begin anytime. According to Rachele, 'A fat bitch is confident, out-spoken, and proud of who she is' (Cateyes 2013b). The ECourse consists of blog posts, web videos, discussion forums, and homework assignments.

Each lesson is intended to educate the participant in an aspect of positive fat ways of being. Lessons in the course include, 'Being fashionable and fat', 'See beauty in other fat bodies', 'Reclaiming the word fat', and 'Being visible and brave'. Individuals engaging in the course are encouraged to consider different ways of perceiving their fatness; revising existing fat identities and living a new kind of fat life. In the course's first lesson, 'You are not giving up', Rachele dismisses the idea that fat women who learn to love and find pride in their bodies are giving up on themselves or on their life. She argues that fat acceptance is not about providing for an excuse for a lifestyle, but a necessary tool to combat fat oppression. In the lesson, the user is given a homework assignment; to write a list of five things they are going to do to make themselves happy. Rachele encourages for the list to contain experiences, actions, and behaviours that users may have previously resisted because of their body size.

Those participating in the course are often prompted to bring others into their journey as well, by blogging their homework, sharing content on Facebook, and engaging in discussions with others in their lives around the topics in the course. There is also a hashtag that participants are encouraged to use (#fatbitchecourse).

In her ECourse, the Nearsighted Owl doesn't simply provide images of a queered fat way of being, she teaches other fats how to engage in queering themselves. Through the coursework, participants are taught to thwart the meanings and associations of fatness put forth by others and develop their own. They construct their own fat identities and learn how to live their fat lives for their own satisfaction.

The Hashtag

Hashtags have become a common way to organise information in cyberspace. A hashtag creates a shared schema; a common understanding that the individuals may use as shorthand in discussion and engagement. Like the #fatbitchecourse hashtag, other tags have been used throughout the fat-o-sphere as a way of bridging information across the web, and promoting the collection of shared experiences. One such hashtag that is successful in the latter is #obeselifestyle.

#obeselifestyle may be found on Twitter, Tumblr, Instagram, and other channels of social media. Like other tags, it allows for the creation of a shared understanding with a single phrase. This particular hashtag is used by fat individuals around the world to embrace and highlight activities that reflect the worst associations of fatness. Searching for #obeselifestyle on Tumblr or Twitter produces pictures and text of food, indulgence, and enjoyment. Some who use the hashtag do so in almost desperation – a throwing up of hands to confess that yes, sometimes, I do the horrid immoral things that others suspect fat people do. Like eat a sundae. Or an entire pizza. Others use the hashtag in glee – reclaiming the allowances their fat identities afford them.

A fun use of the tag may be found on Tumblr, alongside a photo of a 2D donut, and a caption that the user had recently bought a new set of dinner plates. Tossing the #obeselifestyle tag on this post was meant to acknowledge the assumption that of course a fat person would want a plate that looked like a donut. What could be better than gorging oneself on unhealthy food that rests on a vessel that looks like indulgent food? Homer Simpson himself could not have imagined anything better.

The use of the #obeselifestyle tag in reference to food and laziness would seem to some the very opposite of queering fatness. Doesn't it simply reinforce the existing idea that fat people are all lazy and do nothing but eat 'bad' food? In contrast, the use of #obeselifestyle for activities which are explicitly associated with fatness, by fat individuals, is often an act of defying stereotypes. By both embracing and promoting these stereotyped activities, those in the fat-o-sphere are rejecting the negative connotations associated with these activities.

The Colouring Book

Another popular online tag is 'thinspo'. Enter the phrase into a search engine, and it will result in millions of uses of the phrase, tagging material that is supposed to inspire the viewer to strive for thinness. Pictures, memes, blog posts, and other material are tagged as thinspo, and entire Tumblrs and Pinterest boards are filled with said inspiration. The familiar adage, 'Nothing tastes as good as being thin feels' is common, along with other 'inspirational' quotes, pictures of thin bodies, pictures of strong bodies, and an assortment of items that are present to elicit conflicting feelings of shame and pride. They also serve to provide motivation.

Many fat activists have been angered by the use of depictions of fatness under the thinspo tag. Fat bodies, often presented as just pieces of fat bodies, are used to produce a visceral response from the viewer. These pictures are meant to disgust and motivate. Some fat activists have found pictures of themselves used as thinspo (Lutes 2012). Pictures they have uploaded to encourage self-love, reject normative body standards, or inspire confidence in the viewer have been hijacked by users of the thinspo tag. Instead of being used as intended, these pictures have been used as cautionary tales by those lost in 'the fantasy of being thin' (Harding 2007).[5]

To this end, some fat activists began promoting the use of a fatspo tag. By tagging representations of positive fatness as fatspo, they disrupt the discourse on what bodies are aspirational. They attempt to reclaim the narrative back from those who engage in fat shame. One such blogger, Brian Stuart of Red No. 3, actually took this a step further and created the *FATSPO Coloring Book* (Stuart 2013, see also Lorenz 2011's *Fat Ladies in Spaaaaace* coloring book). This book, available on the *FATSPO Coloring Book* Tumblr, is a collection of black and white drawings of inspiring fat individuals. Those interested may download or print the drawings and colour them in as they would an image from a children's colouring book.

Images in the *FATSPO Coloring Book* include celebrities such as Cee Lo Green, Divine, Ashley Fink, and Beth Ditto. Famous faces in the fat-o-sphere appear as well, like Amanda Levitt (Love Your Body Detroit), Kath Read (Fat Heffalump) and the creator, Brian Stuart.

Stuart's *FATSPO Coloring Book* positions fat bodies as aspirational, as things of beauty. This is a rare thing to be had, on or offline. The thinspo tag is meant to inspire fear, guilt, and anxiety; it is meant to help those who believe that

---

5 Harding (2007) suggests that those wrapped up in the fantasy of being thin are clinging to the idea of who they will be, who they will able to become, only once they achieve the magical state of thinness. The fantasy of being thin is often an obstacle for an individual engaging in body acceptance and positivity.

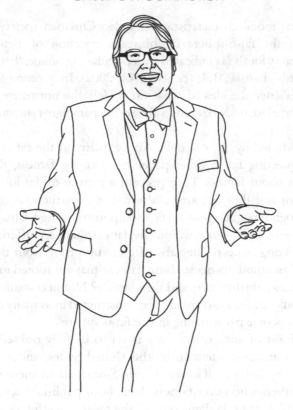

Figure 7.2 Brian Stuart (Red No. 3)
Source: FATSPO Coloring Book.

happiness may only be found through a low BMI. The fatspo tag is meant to inspire acceptance, assurance, and joy; it suggests finding pride in fat ways of being. The *FATSPO Coloring Book* presents an interactive way to queer fat. It flips the idea of thinspo on its head, and suggests that other bodies (in this case, specifically fat bodies) are worthy of celebration and crayons as well.

Is it Useful?

Attitudes toward fatness across much of the world are negative; fat people are thought to be ugly, stupid, lazy, and less likely to succeed in romantic, educational, and professional endeavours (Crandall et al. 2001). But fatness within the fat-o-sphere pushes to be something different. Perhaps fat within the fat-o-sphere suggests a rejection of moral characteristics fat bodies fail to demonstrate. Jutel (2001) argues that fat bodies are read as bodies without discipline and willpower;

both important moral characteristics in Judeo Christian society. Or perhaps fatness within the fat-o-sphere celebrates a rejection of heteronormative, patriarchal, beauty ideals (as indicated by a popular tag online, 'F*ck your fascist beauty standards', harisla 2011; see also Wolf 2002). In queering fatness online, individuals challenge the idea of what fat is, defy the normative roles of, and behaviours related to, body size, and subvert the paradigms surrounding fat and slim bodies.

As demonstrated by the examples above, many in the fat community are engaging in queering fat in cyberspace. By queering fatness, they challenge expected ideas about fatness. They present a picture of fat life that deviates from the norm and they encourage alternative constructions of fat identity. Whether through blogging, posting fashion photos, using hashtags, or various other social media tools, those within the fat-o-sphere are offering a different way of considering fatness. They are offering up proof from their own lives to dispute the assumptions made about fatness that are rooted in essentialism. Fat bodies are lazy, unattractive, and undesirable? Not necessarily[6] in the fat-o-sphere. Fat bodies in the fat-o-sphere are constructed in as many different ways as there are fat people participating in the fat-o-sphere.

The usefulness of such endeavours is yet to be fully realised. The *I Stand* campaign drew national attention in the United States, and Kath Read has been featured in *Australian Women's Weekly*. Stories about these activities, and the work of others who queer fatness, have been published across the world, both online and in print. Perhaps one of the most powerful tools of queering fat within cyberspace is the (un)intentional exposure of others. Many people engage with these activities purposefully, perhaps as part of their own journey in queering fat. Others are unwittingly exposed by friends, family, and those they are following on platforms such as Facebook and Twitter. They are encouraged (forced?) to consider their own perspectives, contemplate a different way of understanding fatness, and learn more about the lives of fat people.

Those engaging in queering fat have lessons to learn as well. A common criticism of much work in the fat-o-sphere is that it represents the voices of a select few in the movement; usually that of white, educated, straight, cis women (Cooper 2008, Peterson 2008, Shannon 2013). Concern has been raised over the lack of representation of those who fall outside of these dominant groups. Those who seek to queer fat within cyberspace would do well to consider the intersectional aspects of any project they embark upon.

---

6 For some in the fat-o-sphere, time has been given to pushing back against the negative associations of laziness or being unattractive. Why be pretty? They argue. Others resist that there is anything wrong with being lazy. What is important is that these fat people are constructing these identities/embodiment/ways of being for themselves; rather than being defined by others.

Through queering fatness, individuals challenge the idea of what it is to be fat, defy the normative roles of, and behaviours related to, body size, and subvert the paradigms surrounding fat and slim bodies. In queering fatness online, those within the fat-o-sphere reject the idea that their bodies are problems that need solutions. They queer what is it to be fat even further by suggesting that fat bodies are to be celebrated. Thus, queering fatness in cyberspace is a very useful tool in fat politics.

References

Aquaporko! The Documentary. 2013. [Film] Directed by Kelli Jean Drinkwater and Anna Helme. Australia: Kelli Jean Drinkwater and Anna Helme.

Butler, J. 1993. *Bodies that Matter: On the Discursive Limits of 'Sex'.* New York: Routledge.

Cateyes, R. 2013a. How to be a fat bitch ECourse #1: You are not giving up. [Online, 1 February] Available at: http://www.nearsightedowl.com/2013/02/how-to-be-fat-bitch-ecourse-1.html [accessed 5 May 2013].

Cateyes, R. 2013b. How to be a fat bitch ECourse #1. [Online, 1 February] Available at: http://www.youtube.com/watch?v=XcQ2uhgqQwI [accessed 5 May 2013].

Cooper, C. 2008. What's fat activism? Working Paper, Department of Sociology. Available at: http://www3.ul.ie/sociology/docstore/workingpapers/wp2008-02.pdf [accessed 15 July 2013].

Cooper, C. and Murray, S. 2012. Fat activist community: A conversation piece. *Somatechnics,* 2(1), 127–138.

Crandall, C.S., D'Anello, S., Sakalli, N., et al. 2001. An attribution-value model of prejudice: Anti-fat attitudes in six nations. *Perspectives of Social Psychology Bulletin,* 27(1), 30–37.

Gibson-Graham, J.K. 1999. Queer(y)ing capitalism in and out of the classroom. *Journal of Geography in Higher Education,* 23(1), 80–85.

Harding, K. 2007. The fantasy of being thin. Shapely Prose. [Online, 27 November] Available at: http://kateharding.net/2007/11/27/the-fantasy-of-being-thin/ [accessed 6 July 2013].

Harding, S. and Kirby, M. 2009. *Lessons from the Fat-O-Sphere: Quit Dieting and Declare a Truce with Your Body.* New York: Penguin.

harisla 2011. F*ck your facist beauty standards. We waste time. [Online, 28 August] Available at: http://wewastetime.wordpress.com/2011/08/28/fuck-your-fascist-beauty-standards/ [accessed 27 August 2013].

Jagose, A. 1996. *Queer Theory.* Dunedin: Otago University Press.

Janmohamed, Z. 2010. Queering Early Childhood Studies: Challenging the discourse of developmentally appropriate practice. *The Alberta Journal of Education Research*, 56(3), 304–318.

Jutel, A. 2001. Weighing health: The moral burden of obesity. *Social Semiotics*, 15(2), 113–125.

Kahn, R. and Kellner, D. 2005. Oppositional politics and the Internet: A critical/reconstructive approach. *Cultural Politics*, 1(1), 75–100.

Lee, H., Learmonth, M. and Harding, N. 2008. Queer(y)ing public administration. *Public Administration*, 86(1), 149–167.

LePeau, L. 2007. Queer(y)ing religion and spiritual: Reflections from difficult dialogues exploring religion, spirituality, and homosexuality. *College Student Affairs Journal*, 26(2), 186–192.

Lohr, K. 2012. Controversy swirls around harsh anti-obesity ads. National Public Radio. [Online, 9 January]. Available at: http://www.npr.org/2012/01 /09/144799538/controversy-swirls-around-harsh-anti-obesity-ads [accessed 1 August 2013].

Lorenz, T.N. 2011. *Fat Ladies in Spaaaaace: A Body-positive Coloring Book*. CreateSpace Independent Publishing Platform.

Lutes, A. 2012. It happened to me: I found my pictures on a thinspo blog. xoJane. [Online, 5 October] Available at: http://www.xojane.com/it-happened-to-me/it-happened-to-me-my-fat-bodys-experience-supported-a-thinspo-bloggers-agenda [accessed 28 August 2013].

NOLOSE. NOLOSE: The revolution just got bigger. [Online] Available at: http://www.nolose.org/index.php [accessed 29 August 2013].

Pausé, C. J. 2012. Live to tell: Coming out as fat. *Somatechnics*, 2(1), 42–56.

Peterson, L. 2008. Intersectionality extends to fat acceptance too! Racialicious. [Online, 24 March] Available at: http://www.racialicious.com/2008/03/24/ intersectionality-extends-to-fat-acceptance-too/ [accessed 30 August 2013].

Read, K. 2013a. The Fat Heffalump. [Online] Available at: http://fatheffalump. wordpress.com/.

Read, K. 2013b. You're not the first to tell a fat person. The Fat Heffalump. [Web blog message, 25 June] Available at: http://fatheffalump.wordpress. com/2013/06/25/youre-not-the-first-to-tell-a-fat-person/ [accessed 1 July 2013].

Robinson, D. 2005. 'Queer(y)ing' gender: Heteronormativity in early childhood education. *Australian Journal of Early Childhood*, 30(2), 19–28.

Rofel, L. 2012. Queer positions: Queer(y)ing Asian Studies. *positions*, 20(1), 183–193.

Sears, J.T. 1999. Teaching queerly: Some elementary propositions, in *Queer(y) ing Elementary Education*, edited by W.J. Letts and J.T. Sears. Lanham, MD: Rowman & Littlefield, 3–14.

Shannon 2013. How to know if you are not doing fat acceptance right. Nudemuse ... daily nattering. [Online, 22 July] Available at: http:// blog.nudemuse.org/2013/07/how-to-know-if-you-are-not-doing-fat. html?zx=3188d1ee6f7cbe74 [accessed 29 August 2013].

Shuai, T., Mozee, G., Tovar, V., et al. 2012. A response to white fat activists by People of Color in the fat justice movement. NOLOSE. [Online] Available at: http://www.nolose.org/activism/POC.php [accessed 31 December 2012].

Stuart, B. 2013. FATSPO Coloring Book. Tumblr. [Online] Available at: http:// FATSPOcoloringbook.tumblr.com/ [accessed 5 August 2013].

Wann, M. 2012. I stand against weight bullying. Tumblr. [Online] Available at: http://istandagainstweightbullying.tumblr.com/ [accessed 30 August 2013].

Warner, M. 1993. Introduction, in *Fear of a Queer Planet*, edited by M. Warner. Michigan: University of Minnesota Press, xxvii.

Wolf, N. 2002 [1991]. *The Beauty Myth: How Images of Beauty are Used Against Women*. New York: HarperCollins.

Chapter 8
Flaunting Fat:
Sex with the Lights On

Jenny Lee

This chapter considers the intersectionality between queer sexuality and a queer fat body. It is framed by my transformation from the culturally expected role of the heterosexual slim woman who engaged in dieting and fat-hatred, to acceptance and celebration of queer sexuality and identity. The stories of that metamorphosis are used to reflect on the nature and reasons for the prejudice, both external and internalised, encountered along that journey. Dieting and shame were my normalised responses to being fat. Refusing to diet and fat acceptance or 'flaunting fat' are a kind of 'coming out' – into a queer identity, without the internalised shame. If mainstream culture portrays fat as an invisible sexuality, and further portrays fat as undesirable, or implies that you're 'stooping' to have sex with someone fat, then how illicit, how queer is it, to be fat and have sex with the lights on?

This chapter is an autoethnographic exploration; part memoir, part commentary, on the state of having a queer body and queer sexuality. My body has slipped in and out of queerness as it has moved from fat to slim and back, until it has settled at fat. This chapter contains narratives of desiring different bodies than are expected and recognises dieting as a kind of fat denial. It addresses the complexities of 'coming out', and the question 'coming out as what?' I used to say I was bisexual because it was easier, but it's not accurate; maybe my queer attractions should be described as butch-trans-friendly-with-fantasies-of-femme-women-with-light-s&m-but-partnered-to-a-gentle-man-with-pot-belly and my queer identity is fat-femme-feminist-with-chipped-nail-polish. The complexities of living with a fat queer identity while the world and loved ones regularly express prejudices against aspects of this identity are explored, culminating in the conclusion that self-acceptance is the first step on a long road to broader acceptance.

During my teenage years, I listened all day to the other students at school, and thought of the ideal, or witty, or interesting thing to say, or occasionally the mean or cutting thing to say, but I rarely said anything. From what I could tell, boys showed no interest in me – I had short hair, was (a bit) pudgy, had few girly interests and was the nerdy dux of year eight. I was almost invisible, except that I was considered smart. I had very little connection to my body, beyond masturbating to my father's foreign film videotapes once everyone was asleep, often involving threesomes, usually followed by a prayer to god asking him to forgive me.

I had crushes on boys I barely spoke to. And my cabbage patch doll, Bazil Grant, got married to my friend Mandy's cabbage patch doll, Beth Janine, and I secretly wished I could brush Mandy's dark silky hair. But I thought that I was ugly and that no one would want me. My mother thought she was ugly too, and it didn't help that my father sometimes commented that she needed to lose weight, while being slim himself. In year 11, I got sick of being me, so I joined the debating team, embarrassed myself by stuttering and turning red, but eventually I was able to talk in public. I lost weight over the summer, with a meal replacement milkshake diet called HerbaLife, and when I came back in year 12 several boys showed interest in me. One asked a friend if I was seeing anyone. My new friends expected me to be happy but I said – they didn't like me when I was fat, so they don't get me now. Instead I went out with a pretty boy (who had silky black 90s hair) from a different school who didn't know what I used to be like. It created a sensation because, by that time, I was appointed school captain (not by popular vote but by interview panel), and no longer invisible, and he was known for throwing ice at Ronald McDonald and setting off car alarms in the western suburb of Keilor Downs.

His best mate, who was a jock at my school, told him I was a nerd, a stiff, and used to be fat, and that he could do better. To his credit, Dan stuck with me. Until I got drunk with a group of friends in a park and was then provoked by a drunken guy, who punched me. I screamed and cried and tried to attack the guy, and when Dan tried to pull me away and keep me safe, I turned on him and called him a bastard. My father had been hitting me for years, and I couldn't handle men controlling me in any way – not even protecting me, or buying me a drink. When Dan broke it off with me I remember that I said, 'I understand. I'm fucked up. It's not my fault, but I understand why you're walking away'. And I knew I couldn't do anything to stop it. But I seemed to be able to observe myself – a future, healthier version of me looking on as the other part of me bumbled through life without the framework to accept myself.

I used to wonder why it took me until I was 26 to come out as queer. I accidentally kissed a girl I loved deeply when I was 20. I went everywhere with Kate, told her everything, bought her beer, fought with her like we were a couple, paid for her to go back to school through TAFE, accepted her sullen sober self and her crazy drunk self. But I insisted I was straight. I got together with a man and eventually walked away from Kate. She didn't stop me. She found a boyfriend on the same day.

When I was 26 I met Jane at a book launch – I told her about my research into the medical management of intersex births and she asked me to read my creative work at a queer event she was organising. I clarified that I wasn't queer and then she put her hand on my arm and I was shot through with sparks. I went home and I thought 'maybe I am queer'. I spent a couple of days feeling as if an alien had abducted and not quite returned me. I wanted to be with a woman, and this wasn't such a shock to my friends.

When she and I did get together, I was afraid to tell my parents – especially my father. When I told him, I cried for a while and then spat it out. He said, 'Is that all? I thought you were going to tell me you had cancer'. So I received acceptance on a certain level. But when my girlfriend started to transition and live as a trans man, my father couldn't say the male name or pronoun. And when my father's puritanical Christian sister told my mum to tell me that I could come to Christmas lunch at her house but my girlfriend couldn't, I didn't go, but my family did. I later forgave my parents and sister but I still haven't forgiven my aunt for excluding my partner. For not accepting me.

I have been judged harshly for being fat and for being bisexual and the feelings associated with both are the same. A steel band tight around my chest, fingers around my throat, a lead ball in my stomach. And then tears.

For a long time I feared judgment more than anything else, and I realised that fear of judgment seems to drive my mother. Whenever there is a special occasion, like Christmas, my mum can be heard throughout the day: I shouldn't be eating this, oh I shouldn't eat this, I shouldn't be eating this, I didn't eat much earlier, but I shouldn't be eating this – as if she says this before anyone else can observe it. I grew up watching her hide and eat food, and I did the same. We hide when we feel shame, when we know we will be judged. When I was about four years old, my mum took me to her fat club. I sat in the corner, at a table, colouring in while they weighed themselves. I looked up to see mum standing up the front, putting on a pig snout attached to elastic. Like a party mask. She and two other women sang the piggy song. This was because she had put on weight that week. When she lost weight she would get a badge to sew onto her blanket.

I was put on my first diet at eight years old after I told my mum, 'I wish I was thinner'. I kept this diet a secret and swore her to secrecy – already I knew to be ashamed. I was hit in bouts of anger by a father who was abused himself as a child, and who also hates fat. I think the fat hatred and the physical abuse got fused together in my mind for a long time – as one and the same thing. My father was bulimic, he used to eat huge bowls of dessert and whipped cream and sometimes he'd throw up. He still compensates for what he eats by exercising excessively and skipping meals. But he's skinny so people think his eating habits are healthy. He watched my sister and me and commented on what we ate, how much we ate, and whether we needed dessert. While I think that people with eating disorders deserve our empathy and love, my father's bulimia and my mother's chronic dieting and bingeing wreaked havoc with my relationship with food.

The lack of medical acknowledgment that someone like my father – slim but not bony – could have an eating disorder, and the usual medical advice to my mother – to lose weight at all costs – reinforced the damaged relationship our family had, and some still have, with food. The attempt to normalise bodies in my family, and to ensure they're not different or fat, led me to conclude that I was ugly. This was before the Internet, before I could Google 'fat naked bodies' and see that my body is, at the very least, similar to a lot of other bodies out there. I have no doubt it also contributed to my fear of speaking to my parents about sexuality, and coming out to them as 'bi'. It may not be this simple, but perhaps I felt that my sexuality wouldn't be accepted because I had always felt that my body was unacceptable, fat and ugly. In my early 20s I got five piercings, in addition to the usual ear piercings, two of which weren't visible to the naked eye. I stretched one of my ear lobes and wore a home-made aluminium cone wrapped in gaffa tape through my ear, and wore jeans that were more rips than denim. I talked obnoxiously about sex and experimentation, and rejected my Anglican schooling as much as I could. My sister had more piercings than me, and several tattoos – each one accompanied by my mother's howls of protest, 'you're ruining your body'. Aesthetics, rebellion, health – it was all really mixed up in our family. But when I told my mother I was seeing a woman, which is how I 'came out', she said that she'd vowed to always support her children if they were gay because her gay cousin had come out to his family and they had rejected him. He had then killed himself. She said she always wished he'd come to her first, before going to his parents, and that maybe he'd still be alive if he had.

I'd never before heard the story of my mother's cousin, and I couldn't help thinking that a vow that paid tribute to him would be to tell his story to your children – and not just if they're gay or queer themselves. But that's only one of the family secrets that I've discovered – trauma and shame and hidden stories are peppered throughout my family history. As I came out, I grieved for this dead family member. Soon after that my mother reassured another relative that it wasn't her fault her son is gay – that she thinks it runs in the family.

There was a time when I didn't acknowledge that I am attracted to women. (I want to write 'some women' as it seems strange to state 'I am attracted to women' or 'I am attracted to men and women'). Then there was a time where I could acknowledge that I was attracted to women – if I was drunk. Then came the time where I was attracted to a particular woman and decided to accept that I am bisexual … or something queer. I say 'decided to accept' because I think acceptance is a decision that crops up daily or weekly or erratically, and has to be made over and over again. I dated Jane, who told me about her past attempt at binding her breasts and chopping up dresses as a child. I decided to accept – when he asked to be called James – that he wanted to change his identity and perhaps his body. On one level I accepted that he should be who he felt he wanted to be, but on another level, perhaps I related to a desire to change the body to fit your idea of who you are. At the time, in my mind, fat was ugly, fat represented flaws and laziness and not being good enough, fat represented my father's rejection. So of course I wanted to be slim. In some ways, my relationship with my body was very different to James's relationship with his body. As far as I observed, his desire for change included shedding other people's expectations that he would conform to his allocated female gender and upbringing, whereas my desire for change was about conforming to what I thought a woman should be.

Perhaps because so many anti-fat messages are framed by health policy, we didn't ask the question: what could be wrong with trying to lose weight? I encouraged James to bind his breasts, and meet others who felt a similar way, and he encouraged me to meet my own queer friends, and embrace my femmeness rather than cutting my hair and losing the skirts. I organised 'Femme Fever', a spoken word event, for the Melbourne Midsumma Queer Festival and there were heels and lipstick flashes – and also butch women – everywhere. But still I was counting calories and buying 'flattering' clothes. All the while, James, like the partner before and the partner after, loved my fat body. Despite this, I was conforming to my father's ideal – thin, thin, thin. Yet, while I accepted James's transforming identity, and he accepted and loved my fat body, I was on Weight Watchers, and neither of us had the knowledge or language at the time, to say 'you need to accept your fat body'.

I think back to that amazing period of coming out. But coming out as what? As sort-of bisexual, but maybe rhi-sexual would be better, after the rhizome – a messy root with many branches that theorists Deleuze and Guattari discuss in *A Thousand Plateaus*.[1] And my 'girlfriend' came out publically too – a year into our relationship – as a trans man. I came out as femme in what seemed a rather unfriendly environment to femmes. But I was still 'in the closet', if we see dieting as a kind of fat denial. Dieting suppressed the body I should have had. And my body kept trying to come out as fat – over and over. When the dieting wasn't sustainable and my hunger took over. At the time I was letting loose those sexual hungers I'd kept in bondage for years, but I was still suppressing my hunger and appetite to get the body I thought I should have. When I realised, sometime around 28 years of age, eight years ago now that I was still bingeing at night when my Weight Watchers points had run out, albeit on roast vegetables sprayed with olive oil, and dry Vitawheats, I did some looking around. Now I wonder if bingeing is the right word – I was downright

---

1 Deleuze, G. and Guattari, F. (1997). *A Thousand Plateaus: Capitalism and Schizophrenia.* B. Massuni (trans.) Minneapolis: University of Minnesota Press.

hungry. Maybe 'extra-hungry' eating at night is more the word for it. I attended a moderate eating group at Swinburne University and learnt about giving up dieting and listening to my body – which was a good first step. I still wanted to lose weight, and the program didn't quite make the link to fat acceptance for me. Sometime after this, I saw a dietician who had worked with a moderate eating programme, and still she suggested I might need some boundaries to control my eating. I had resumed eating larger amounts of high calorie foods, and she said that, if we consider cows grazing in a field, with no fences, I was straying outside the invisible boundaries, and we needed to put some fences in, or I'd stray too far. I believed her at the time, but actually, my eating only became 'moderate' and 'normal' when I truly allowed myself to eat whatever I wanted whenever I wanted it, without restriction. If she had asked me how I felt about butter, chips, ice-cream, and chocolate, she would have discovered my fear surrounding those foods and their power over me. They don't have that power over me anymore because I can have them if I want them, and, in true rebellion, like-a-girl-who-plays-hard-to-get, I only wanted them in excess when I thought I couldn't have them. Just like when I was four years old, eating lollies behind my dad's back until I was sick. At 28, I hadn't truly found my voice yet and it took me years more to do so. But that was understandable, considering there was a time when I barely spoke.

I now believe I have a queer identity and a queer body. It's more complicated than saying all fat people are queer. They're not. Am I right to say that fat people who diet, hate their bodies and engage in normalised shame for having a fat body are not queer? And that those of us who accept or flaunt our fat, who have sex with the lights on, are queer? Or are fat bodies essentially queer in our Western culture because they are not considered 'normal', not displayed as attractive? It seems easier to pose these questions than to answer them.

I have been judged and shamed more widely for being fat than I have for being 'bisexual', but part of that might be because I am a cisgendered femme woman and I (think I) often pass as heterosexual. The judgment for being fat spans from being oinked at on the street, to women in boutique shops looking down upon me, to medical specialists dissecting what I eat and hunting for what I'm doing wrong, to my own father watching what I ate when I was a teen. But all western fat people experience the institutional prejudice – the media, the medical establishment, the government, the public health messages. The world wants fat people to disappear, to become thin.

Over the years I have struggled with taking the emphasis off weight loss and putting it on health and well-being instead. A hospital dietician that was allocated to me recently to assist with a dietary issue – not 'obesity' – advised me to go to the gym five times a week. My twice a week at the gym and walking my dog three to four times a week were not good enough for her (for the dog lovers – my partner walks him on other days). She told me that walking my dog as a form of exercise wasn't a good idea, because dogs slow down to sniff things and pee, and your heart rate goes down. Therefore, it's not effective exercise for weight loss. She didn't think about the fact that I could fit a dog walk into my life more easily than the gym, that it was the only time I got any sunshine and fresh air, that I laughed at my dog's antics, his waggy tail and rolling on grass and playing with me or other dogs. That it is good for my mental and physical health. She didn't ask how long I walked him for or find out that he likes to run on the oval, so I often have to walk fast or jog to keep up with him. I feel confident that a thin person seeing her for dietary advice would not have received this advice. Her focus was heart rate and weight loss, and there was no room for my individual needs, even when I told her, with a shaky voice, that I could pick up any newspaper and read about obesity, that the weight focus wasn't useful for me. She persisted in hunting for issues with my diet – and located one when I told her I cook a Thai curry once every three or four weeks. She asked if I use low-fat coconut milk and I said no, I use full-cream coconut milk. I got a whole speech about that. Her prejudice meant that I didn't find out any new information that could help me. She tried to shame me into conforming. Her words echoed in my mind for several weeks afterwards. As I took a bite of chocolate, I'd think, 'fuck you'. I didn't conform but I struggled to throw off the shroud of shame she draped me with. Sometimes I do think things would be easier or I'd fit in better or be considered more beautiful if I did lose weight. That's hard to avoid. But to be in an environment where to be fat is okay, with no judgment – is important.

James and I broke up around eight years ago. When I met my current partner, Nick, who is a heterosexual male, seven years ago, I started to think of myself as an invisible queer. I think I pass as a straight woman unless I tell people I am bi or queer, although lots of people tend to think all outspoken women are lesbians, so I can't be sure. I've started to realise that some queers have to come out, time and time again, and that gives us certain privileges – to not have to come out in front of a bigot or on a train late at night with a scary fellow traveller, for starters. This is where clothes and accessories can sometimes indicate identity – perhaps I could show I am queer with a buzz cut, and a bright tight-fitting top to show off my fat. I'd be a defiant fat lesbian. But I'm an introvert and I like the Melbourne aesthetic of grey, black and splashes of red. I like being femme but I don't tend to show off my body. I've never chosen a cleavage top on purpose (sometimes I can't help it if I lean over – these things can catch food if I'm not careful). I'm comfortable, mostly, in bathers, and I strip off easily for my massage therapist, so my self-acceptance levels are much better than they were. But I've questioned whether I'm betraying the fat movement to wear a loose silk top or all black – or floppy trackies to the gym. Shouldn't I be sporting lycra at the gym and bright colours when I go to the pub? No. I have heels and lingerie just for the bedroom, and I leave the lights on, but I'm not really a flaunter. I admire the fat burlesque crew in VaVaBoomBah, and I love some of the fat nude photography I've seen by Georgia Laughton and Substantia Jones, but I doubt I'll be posing. I accept that I am an introverted fat activist, who rehearses before speaking about fat issues in public. I accept that people don't know I'm queer until they talk to me. I accept that some days I wish I was thin, just so life could be easier, before I take a few deep breaths and accept all over again that I am fat.

It's only been since I've met fellow fatties and attended 'fat' events that I have settled into my body properly, that I've had the confidence to talk back to anti-fat doctors, and to tell my dad about Health at Every Size. My relationship with my body has become celebratory at times, especially when watching Aquaporko; the fat synchronised swimming group, and when chatting with a fat reading group I started with the support of Victoria University. Engaging with other fat writers, artists and activists has made all the difference.

I'm fat/queer. I never asked myself why I am attracted to multiple genders, so although there might be reasons I am fat, I'm going to stop trying to figure them out. Who cares if someone is fat because they like butter on everything, or because they carry an undiscovered gene, or because they grew up with a binge eater and a bulimic, or because they just are. I've looked at it from so many angles, and it hasn't changed shape. And, lately, I haven't really changed shape that much either.

Chapter 9

Queering the Linkages and Divergences: The Relationship between Fatness and Disability and the Hope for a Livable World

Zoë Meleo-Erwin

May 6, 2010 marked the 18th anniversary of 'International No Diet Day', an event devoted raising awareness about anti-fat discrimination, exposing the inefficacy of dieting, celebrating a diversity of body sizes, and other related goals. On that date, fat activist[1] and fat studies scholar Charlotte Cooper (2010a) blogged about her experiences with the British group 'Dietbreakers' that began the tradition. In her post on her blog *Obesity Timebomb*, Cooper highlights the contributions Dietbreaker's founder Mary Evans Young made for the fat activist movement. However as the piece develops, she then raises significant critique of the group's structure and tactics. In particular, Cooper notes that she disagreed with the assimilationist stance that Dietbreakers and other early 1990s fat activists groups took by seeking mainstream acceptance of fat bodies and yet conceding that the very large would still benefit from weight loss (presumably for health related reasons). What is of interest in Cooper's post for my purposes here is her mention of what remains a sticking point for size diversity activism today – the contentious relationship between fatness, health, and disability.

---

1 While 'fat activism' and 'size diversity' are somewhat different framings, they both share the same focus on fighting fat-phobia and promoting the social, political, and cultural inclusion of a diversity of body sizes and shapes, and are thus used interchangeably here to avoid redundancy. Following Cooper (2010b) it is important to note that fat activism, which is entwined with the academic discipline of fat studies, is not a coherent social movement, per se, and rather can be seen as the diverse collection of activist groups, organisations, events, clubs, researchers, websites, Internet forums, legal actions, bloggers, zine makers, amongst others, that at a very minimum agree upon the need to challenge anti-fat stigma and stereotypes.

The Tricky Politics of Fatness, Health and Disability

The medical, public health, and media sectors steadfastly maintain that fatness, or 'obesity' in its medicalised term, is an epidemic disease that threatens population health and well-being.[2] In the United States, the CDC, NIH, and Office of the Surgeon General all point to the complex potential interaction between behavioural, genetic, and environmental causes of fatness. Despite this, the role of the individual in taking charge of zier health, fitness, and weight loss is commonly emphasised in national public health information, and popularly fatness is generally considered to be the fault of the fat.[3] Given that fatness is attributed to a lack of self-control and will power, anti-fat sentiment has both strong moral undertones and overtones. In response, much of size diversity activism has been devoted to challenging this purported relationship between fatness, health, and morality.

Fat activism often highlights the failure of diets to produce durable weight loss and the lack of conclusive evidence either linking fatness with increased morbidity and mortality, or dieting with improved health outcomes (cf. Harding and Kirby 2009, Wann 1999). Further, many fat studies scholars have suggested that the war against obesity constitutes more of a 'moral panic' and a lucrative war on fat people than a legitimate strategy to improve public health (cf. Campos et al. 2006, Herndon 2005). As Kirkland's (2008) work demonstrates, a strategy taken by some fat activists is to highlight the fact that one can eat healthfully and exercise but still be fat. Yet in doing so, fat activism has risked pathologising those whose fatness can be more directly attributed to behaviour – specifically a lack of physical activity and/or to particular eating habits – thus leaving in place culturally dominant logics about normalcy, health, difference, and rights (Kirkland 2008). This is a quandary given that size diversity groups do not seek to paint some fat people, particularly the very fat, as 'worthy' of discrimination and yet cannot escape questions about the linkages between size, health, and disability.

Responding to this issue, some fat activists and fat studies scholars (Cooper 1997, Kinzel 2008) have attempted to decentre issues of health and foreground

---

2 Following fat studies, I use 'fat' here not in the commonly held pejorative sense, but rather as a neutral descriptor of embodiment such as 'tall' or 'brown-eyed'. The term 'obesity' is used when describing the ways in which fatness has become medicalised (cf. Chang and Christakis 2002, Jutel 2006, Shwartz 1986) and is treated as both a disease and an epidemic by medical, public health, media, and popular sectors.

3 Puhl and Brownell (2003: 216) state: '… it appears that this bias remains strong even in the face of a large prevalence of obese adults and children, and despite contradictory research evidence that demonstrates the limited success of long-term weight loss'.

connections with disability rights. For such individuals, the focus of size diversity activism should not be whether or not one can be fat and healthy but rather, fat activism should pose the question: 'why should health status or physical ability be the basis for discrimination?' Fat activist blogger and author Lesley Kinzel's November 2008 post 'Embracing the Morbid' is illustrative in this regard. She writes:

> There are lots of people fatter than me. There are people who are fatter and in better shape, there are people who are less fat and in worse condition. There are individual fat people with a far broader range of physical abilities than me, and individual fat people whose range of abilities is much narrower. There are also fat people whose abilities are simply different, and neither better nor worse. Choose a weight from the air, and I'll bet you real money that I can line you up ten people at that weight with dramatically different bodies and experiences and lives. It's okay to not always be the Good Fat Person. I don't have to represent the best of fat people everywhere, and neither do you. I don't have to defend my choices. They're no one's business but my own.

Kinzel and others thus make critical linkages between fat activism and disability rights by challenging the idea that fat bodies and disabled bodies are flawed and worthy of discrimination. Along these lines, some fat studies scholars (Ampramor 2010, Cooper 1997) have specifically asked the question 'does fatness belong under the umbrella of disability?'

Following Ampramor (2010), Cooper (1997) and others, I first trace the connections and divergences made between fatness and disability in fat studies and Disability Studies. In doing so, I pay specific attention to the application of the 'social model' of disability to fatness. I then suggest that fat activism and fat studies should consider critiques of the social model made by disability scholars and activists. Specifically, fat activism and fat studies should take note of the ways in which the social model fails to challenge healthist norms of embodiment. Rather than asking 'does fatness belong under the umbrella of disability', I propose that a queering of both disability and fatness provides a stronger critique of neoliberal healthism and may allow for fat and disability activists and scholars to make strategic alliances while simultaneously preserving the unique needs and focuses of each individual movement.[4]

---

4 It is important to note that while any given body may be both fat and disabled, in this chapter I examine fat and disabled movements (inclusive of fat and disability studies), which are distinct from one another.

Fatness as Disability?

Disability rights activists and scholars routinely note that the term 'disabled' covers a wide range of categories (including psychiatric, cognitive, and physical disabilities as well as chronic illnesses), which, at first face, may seem to have little in common with one another. However as Garland-Thomson (1997), Linton (1998), and others have argued, what unites these categories is the meaning made of them and its impact. In the 1970s, British Activists in the Union of the Physically Impaired Against Segregation (UPIAS) challenged what they termed the 'medical model' of disability, or the framing of impaired bodies by the medical and rehabilitation sectors as fundamentally flawed and in need of correcting or curing. In its stead they posed the 'social model'. This model differentiated between 'impairments', seen as located in the body, and 'disability', which was defined as the ways in which the social and built environment create barriers for those with impairments by reflecting and privileging the able-bodied. The social model held that what united individuals with a diverse range of impairments was the common experience of marginalisation and exclusion. Abelism was thus held to be an oppression and disability rights was the political strategy that would dismantle the barriers to full inclusion. A similar model developed in the United States wherein disabled people were seen to be a minority group and inclusion was framed as a civil rights issue (Fine and Asch 1988, Shakespeare and Watson 2002).[5]

Finding inspiration in the social model and making linkages with fatness, Cooper (1997), in an early fat studies article, asked 'can a fat woman call herself disabled?' Cooper noted that like the impaired body, the fat body is a site of medical intervention with fatness held to be a pathological physiological state in need of correcting. Both groups, she continued, are stigmatised and discriminated against; face barriers in fully accessing the built environment; are simultaneously hyper visible and invisible, and are pressured to undergo normalising procedures, which, themselves often cause physiological and psychological harm.[6] Echoing many disability rights advocates who have

---

5 Both the social and minority models stressed the importance of addressing 'the social, structural, and psychological situation of people with disabilities' regardless of whether or not individuals identified as 'disabled' or shared a political consciousness (Fine and Asch 1988: 7).

6 A further commonality worth mentioning is that fat activism and scholarship, as with disability rights and scholarship, has begun as a largely middle class, white, movement (Kirkland 2008, O'Toole 2004, Shakespeare 1999) despite the fact that people of colour and working class and poor people are more likely to be fat (and disabled) than are white and middle class people (Centers for Disease Control 2009, Olkin 1999). Unlike disability rights, however, fat activism is largely lead by women and is far more queer in many facets. For more on the ways in which fat and disability

argued that impairment is a part of human variation but under a system of oppression has become a category of social and political significance (Linton 1998, Garland-Thomson 2005), Cooper states: '… I regard fatness as a normal state of being, neither healthier nor less healthy than any other body shape or size, and part of the amazing diversity of body types' (35).

While she states that she considers fat embodiment in a fat-phobic environment to be disabling, Cooper also notes that there are important differences between fat and disabled groups that must be elucidated. Notably, fat people do not share a history of institutionalisation with disabled people;[7] fat people, in general, do not experience the life-long engagement with medical processionals that those born with disabilities do, and fat people are often blamed for their fatness and are therefore the objects of scorn unlike disabled people, who are usually seen the objects of pity.[8] While these differences may pull the two groups apart, the internalisation of stereotypes by each group about the other may cause further separation. Cooper suggests that disability rights advocates, having been raised in fat-phobic environments and possibly having internalised stereotypes about fat people, may reject them, seeing their cause as trivial in comparison and their bodily state an elective one. Fat activists who use disability rights framing and language may also be seen as co-opting and colonising the work of disability rights. And finally, fat people, if they have internalised the medical model of disability, may not wish to identify as disabled and instead may focus on refuting the belief that fatness is or leads to a state of ill health. Though she does not conclusively determine that fatness belongs under the umbrella of disability, Cooper argues that these differences, while important, 'need not threaten political unity' as 'people with many different kinds of impairments have come together as disabled and this mixture has forged a rich and diverse culture' (40).

Twelve years later in the same journal, *Disability & Society*, Aphramor (2009) took up Cooper's question. She opens her article with a rhetorical question, 'For if disability is understood as the interplay of aspects of (possible) impairment and social exclusion premised on medicalised assumptions of pathology or

---

rights activism and scholarship may unwittingly reproduce race and class privilege and therefore remain irrelevant to those most directly affected by fat phobia and ableism, see Shuai (2008) and Bell (2006). See also: http://www.nolose.org/activism/POC.php.

7 However see Solovay (2000) who documents cases of the forced institutionalisation of fat children for the purposes of weight loss.

8 Kirkland (2008) argues that, unlike disability, fatness is seen as mutable and voluntary, both popularly and legally. Because of this, the solution to anti-fat stigma is held to be weight loss, not legal protections. However, she suggests that fat politics – if it can move beyond defensive anti-discrimination arguments that are based on health status – has the potential to challenge linkages between bodily difference, choice (or lack thereof) and rights.

deficiency, how is fatness, invariably diagnosed as 'overweight/obese' [sic] and read as the disease 'obesity', not disabling?' (897, parenthetical statements are Aphramor's). Aphramor makes interesting linkages between fatness and psychiatric disabilities, noting that both have been the targets of a 'plethora of harmful quasi-scientific interventions' (900). This comparison is compelling in that slimness and mental health are both highly elastic categories and increasingly we are all encouraged to take action to ensure them (Rose 2006).[9] Noting that fat individuals are not necessarily disabled, she nevertheless argues that the promotion of thinness by medical professionals is, in part, based on abelist assumptions. Aphramor further suggests that, despite the differences between the two groups, considering them together invites new openings for social transformation and she advocates that health practitioners, such as herself, take up Oliver's (1999: 5) claim to 'address the political dimensions of their work' in regard to both disability and fatness.

Although some disability studies theorists discuss fatness as falling within the category of disability, this does not appear to be common. However, Herndon (2002) and Garland-Thomson (2005) have discussed the relationship between the two at length. Herndon (2002) suggests that there are many connections between the social construction and social reception of fat and disabled bodies. Both groups, she argues, offer different narratives of life than those usually provided in medical and popular accounts, and thus disrupt normative accounts of disability and fatness; both groups are accused of driving up national health care costs; both fat and deaf people are encouraged and often pressured to

---

9 Given that the World Health Organization predicts that mental illness, particularly depression, will rank 2nd in the global burden of disease by 2020 (http://www.who.int/mental_health/advocacy/en/Call_for_Action_MoH_Intro.pdf) and frames obesity as a global epidemic (http://www.who.int/dietphysicalactivity/en/index.html), the treatment and prevention of mental illness and fatness are not merely a public health priorities but highly lucrative businesses. Aphramor notes that the US diet industry was worth over $35 billion in 2006 and Reuters reports that in 2009, US sales of antipsychotics and antidepressants alone garnered 24.5 billion (see: http://www.reuters.com/article/idUSTRE6303CU20100401). In that these figures are unlikely to include the profits from weight loss surgeries, gym memberships, supplements, doctor's visits or therapy sessions, they are a vast underestimate of the total worth of the weight loss and mental health industries. Further, the 'obesity epidemic' has ironically become profitable for the very food and beverage industries that are seen by some public health scholars (Nestle 2000, Schwartz and Brownell 2007) as having majorly contributed to the obesity epidemic in the first place. These industries have not only marketed certain of their products as 'whole grain' or 'low fat' while continuing to produce the standard versions, but have waged a significant public relations campaign promoting exercise over diet as a cause of obesity and healthful eating as a 'choice'. For more on this, see Herrick (2009).

adopt normalising surgeries; both groups have politicised their experiences, and finally both groups provoke anxiety by highlighting the fluidity and transitory nature of the body.

Garland-Thomson (2005: 1560) argues that one of the goals of feminist disability studies is to trouble and politicise 'ideological concepts such as health, disease, normalcy, cure and treatment'. She notes that such a perspective involves a consideration of those bodies that are not classically considered disabled and argues for the importance of considering 'appearance impairments'. To this end, she notes: 'Perhaps the most common bodily form vehemently imagined as failed or incorrect is the fat body' (1581). Those with appearance impairments, such as fatness, are often subjected to bodily disciplining through surgical and other normalisation interventions, and pressures to undergo such procedures bespeak 'modernity's fierce drive to limit human variation … and its intolerance toward contradictory bodies' (1580). Garland-Thomson further notes that while fatness is always an appearance impairment, it is also at times a physical one. In this sense, she argues, fatness is a disability issue.

Beyond the Social Model: Taking a Further Lesson from Disability Studies and Activism

Although they might be in the minority, it is clear that some scholars and activists are making critical linkages between fatness and disability. Given that fat activism and scholarship are arguably younger and less developed than their disability rights and studies counterparts, we might ask how the latter might inform the former. In her work Cooper (1997) illustrates the utility of the social model for fat activism and studies. She states: 'Being fat is considered a personal 'problem', a medical affliction which can be 'cured' by weight loss … In contrast, a social model reframes our experiences of self-hatred and stigma as a public and political issue, and suggests that the problem lies within social constructions of prejudice and not in our bodies' (39). This perspective can be seen as common within much of fat activism and studies (cf. Campos 2004, Wann 1999). As with disability, the social model has been of great asset to fat activism. In addition to helping to reframe self-hatred, as Cooper (1997) notes, such a perspective has helped to create community and galvanise political action.[10]

On first face, the application of the social model to fat activism seems entirely positive. However, despite the many clear benefits of this model within disability rights (e.g. the development of a social and political identity, the creation of

---

10 Cf. the National Association for the Advancement of Fat People: http://www.naafaonline.com/.

community, and the opening up of employment, education, community based housing, transportation, access to more of the built environment, etc.), it has increasingly become the object of critique within disability rights and studies. Given the linkages between fatness and disability, I suggest it is imperative that fat activism and studies take note of these critiques.

Within the social sciences and humanities, the body has become a site of scholarly investigation, and interest lies not only in the ways in which the body can be seen to be discursively produced, but ontologically 'enacted' (Moll 2007) and phenomenologically experienced (Crossley 1995). The social model differentiates between impairment (based in the body) and disability (barriers within the social model that exclude people with impairments from full participation). The main thrust of contemporary disability studies critiques (which differ from one another) is that this model reproduces the 'disembodied Cartesian subject' (Hughes and Paterson 1997, Shakespeare and Watson 2002); misses the ways in which impairment and disability, like the body and social environment, are dialectically related (Shakespeare and Watson 2002); ignores the experiential aspect of impairment (Hughes 1999), and is based on the experiences of the 'healthy disabled' but ignores the experiences of those with chronic and progressive diseases (Morris 2001, Wendell 2001). I briefly review these critiques below.

In separating the body from the social and built environment, what has been referred to as the 'strong version' of the social model (Shakespeare and Watson 2002) reproduces the Cartesian mind/body dualism by suggesting that the body is natural, pre-social, and pre-cultural (Hughes 1999, Shakespeare and Watson 2002) and that impairments are best managed in the private and perhaps medical spheres (Thomas 2004). In this sense, the social model 'concedes that impairment is a disfigurement and therefore accepts the medico-aesthetic distinction between valid and invalid bodies. This position actually lends legitimacy to accounts of impairment that are shaped by notions of tragedy and pity' (Hughes 1999: 168). In contradistinction to the impairment/disability dualism, Shakespeare and Watson (2002) see the two as dynamically intertwined. Hughes and Paterson (1997: 329) argue that impairment is more than a biological or medical issue 'it is both an experience and a discursive construction'. They further argue that not only is impairment is entangled with culture and social structure, but that oppression is both political and embodied as pain and suffering.

Many disability scholars argue that impairment, and particularly its relationship to pain, is part of daily experience and cannot be ignored in disability rights or studies (Shakespeare and Watson 2002). The fact that it has been has meant that many disabled people cannot easily recognise themselves within the social model (Landsman 2009) and therefore disability studies and activism may not be seen as highly relevant to a number of disabled people (Shakespeare and Watson

1996). Wendell (2001) notes that disability activists have fought being identified with illness and cures for fears that such identifications would contribute to further medicalisation and discrimination. Nevertheless, she continues, many disabled people are in fact sick. She therefore notes that disabled people are both healthy and unhealthy and suggests that disability studies and activism, as currently constituted, better reflects the perspectives, needs, and experiences of the former at the expense of the latter.

Shakespeare and Watson (2002) and Wendell (2001) argue that disability studies and rights must instead make room for the 'unhealthy disabled' (a category Wendell notes is highly elastic) by allowing their experiences to openly acknowledged, discussed, and accommodated. This includes the recognition of the fact that those with chronic illnesses, particularly those that wax and wane, are often treated with suspicion and blame in a way that other disabled people are not. Morris (2001) worries that if the disability rights and studies does not make room for such perspectives, non-disabled bodied people will continue to suggest that their lives are not worth living.

To this end, Shakespeare and Watson (2002) state that we must recognise that different impairments have different individual and social implications. They further argue disability rights and studies are capable of arguing for both the end to social barriers and for assistance with and even prevention of certain impairments. An 'adequate social theory of disability', would therefore include, 'all the dimensions of disabled people's experiences: bodily, psychological, cultural, social, political, rather than claiming that disability is either medical or social' (Shakespeare and Watson 2002: 19). Wendell (2001: 18) contends that an expanded notion of disability politics must recognise that: 'Some unhealthy disabled people, as well as some healthy people with disabilities, experience physical or psychological burdens that no amount of social justice can eliminate'. She further argues for a multiplicity of versions of disability pride, including those which acknowledge that 'suffering is part of some valuable ways of being' (2001: 31).[11]

I want to suggest that fat studies and activism must also acknowledge that while the social model can be a 'powerful organising principle, a rallying cry,

11 Notably, 'disability justice' activism, which is predominantly led by people of colour, low income people, women, and LGBTQ people, differentiates itself from the disability rights movement through its focus on both intersectionality and interdependence. As Mingus (2010) notes, disability justice moves away from an equality model, based on seeking rights and accommodations, to a form of activism that seeks to dismantle the social, political-economic, and cultural conditions which make inaccessibility and oppression possible in the first place. Unsurprisingly, given this framework, disability justice work has been much more inclusive and reflective of those with chronic illnesses.

and a practical tool' (Thomas 2004), fat studies and activism must similarly acknowledge its limitations. In essence, the social model fails to challenge neoliberal healthist norms around embodiment and thus shifts but does not dismantle the borders and boundaries around who is seen as deserving of political recognition and redress. I argue that fat activism must allow for a more complex and nuanced understanding of fatness that includes not only resistance and celebration, but suffering, pain and even desires and measures taken to be less fat. Such a focus would allow fat activists to acknowledge that there are 'healthy fat people' and 'unhealthy fat people', and that in some cases, illness and disability are strongly associated with fatness. Fat activists could continue to argue that fatness is a form of human variation, that dieting does not produce durable weight loss, and that it may be in fact be harmful, while also agreeing that the complex and still contentious relationship between weight, health, illness, impairment, and stigma might mean that fat people make greater demands on health care systems, as is the case with some disabled people.

Fat activists might ask the question 'Why is it ok to say we can be denied our rights as citizens because it costs too much?' (Mairs 1996, quoted in Morris 2001). Such a focus allows for dismantling neoliberal and healthist notions of citizenship as tied to the low-risk and risk-adverse rational subject[12] and instead makes room for counter-notions that allow for difference, interdependence, and even vulnerability and choice (Kirkland 2008). In addition, it brings into sharp relief the dangers of using, as Kirkland (2008: 416) argues, 'the 'master's tools' to construct [our] own plausible inclusion'. Ultimately, this framework may provide a way out of the tricky politics of health, disability, and fat that currently constrain some elements of fat activism and scholarship (Kirkland 2008). By moving outside this terrain we may shift our focus onto the ways in which concepts such as health, illness, normalcy, pathology, and cure are ideological in nature (Garland-Thomson 2005, Kirkland 2008) and examine how they 'function both as norms and as practices of regulation and control' (Schildrick and Price 1996).

---

12 Under what Foucault (1990) described as a bio political mode of governance, great focus is placed on health and vitality of the population and systems of measurement, classification, ordering, and identification allow intervention at the mass level. These systems and interventions effectively produce some bodies as normal and others as pathological. Population-level statistics can, in this sense, be seen to constitute a technology of risk, or a 'way of managing the individualization of people in aggregate classes, through the calculation of the probabilities of certain events and the application of such calculations to individual people' (Kirkland 2003: 46). See also Peterson (2003).

Queering the Linkages and Divergences

Warner (1999) and Kelly (2002) suggest that the notion of 'queer' moves us outside the politics of shame and toward an ethos in which we neither deny the complicated, messiness of the body nor are tempted to redefine these characteristics as normal as a strategy of stigma-management. By resisting the naturalness of sexuality and gender, queer theory calls into question the legitimacy of all identity labels, exposing identity's historically contingent and socially constructed and socially produced nature. Following Hahn (1988), Herndon (2002), and (McRuer 2006), I argue that both fat bodies and disabled bodies are *queer modes of embodiment* in that they elicit great anxiety through the disruption of norms about how bodies are supposed to look and how they are supposed to function. Ultimately this anxiety can be seen to arise from the fact that these forms of embodiment unsettle the belief in the fixity of the body and point to its fluidity (McRuer 2006). In an era of neoliberalism, in which individuals are believed to have a personal and national responsibility for maintaining their own health, particularly in regard to acting pre-emptively acting to stave off that for which they might be at risk[13] (Rose 2006), non-normative modes of embodiment remind us that this is ultimately a losing battle. Bodily normativity can thus be seen as an unstable category that must be constantly performed because it is always, in effect, failing (McRuer 2006). Or in the words Shildrick and Price (1996: 106), the body always exceeds control and in this way 'the specter of the other lurks within the selfsame'. Because of this, the anxiety produced by the constant resolidification of bodily normativity requires non-normative forms of embodiment[14] to shore up categories of normativity (Garland-Thomson 1997, McRuer 2006).

Queering the concept of fat, as others have done with disability (McRuer 2006), allows us to decentre scholarship and activism that focuses on expanding the notion of 'normal' to include us. For the concept of 'normal' is malleable and can change when conditions demand this (Tremain 2008). And without question, 'normal' is a seductive, if not compulsory category, particularly for those who find themselves relegated to a state of pathology. As Parens (2006)

---

13 While normality is a technique of power through which individuals make decisions that make them more governable in the present, risk is a normalising technique 'aimed at governing (managing and controlling) the future' (Waldschmidt 2008: 197).

14 Importantly, this relation is never outside of white supremacy, classism, sexism, cissexism and other forms of oppression but in fact depends on and is produced through them. Thus, those fat and disabled bodies which are designated as most abject and which are made to do the most work to shore up categories of normativity are always already the bodies of people of colour, the poor and working class, women, transgender people, and other marginalised groups.

reminds us, the desire to be normal is the desire for recognition, community, respect and love. It is therefore difficult to chastise those who seek assimilation either on the bodily level through normalising surgeries and practices or on the collective level as the end point of a social movement. However the trouble with normal, as Kelly (2002) reminds us, is that it can require us to hide differences that are salient to us and can leave behind those who are least able or willing to measure up, for norms are not only descriptive but prescriptive (Davis 2006, Kittay 2006). What's more, by distancing ourselves from those who least approximate normalcy, we may reinforce hierarchies along the lines of gender, race, class, sex, gender identity, and other modes of identification. Thus a queer focus might instead look to expose 'the failure of those norms to ever fully contain or express their ideal standards' (Shildrick and Price 1996: 107) and to both trouble and disrupt difference from becoming translated into structures of privilege, oppression, and domination (Baynton 2008). It further allows us to make social and political those issues that heretofore we had relegated to the realm of private, such as suffering, pain, and ambivalence without conceding that our lives are not worth living and that we are not deserving of justice.

A 'Queercrip consciousness', in McRuer and Wilkerson's (2003: 7) words, 'resists containment and imagines other, more inventive, expansive and just communities'. To this end, I suggest queering our framework may allow for strategic alliances between fat and disability activism and studies as part of a broad-based movement for social justice, while preserving the unique focus and needs of each.[15] I believe it is important to make such strategic connections in the realm of scholarship and activism and yet retain some separate focus for in the end, despite our commonalities, fat people and disabled groups are not always treated the same way nor do we necessarily have the same needs.

In order to make such alliances, it is important for disability studies and activism to challenge the notions that fat is mutable and voluntary and therefore unworthy of political consideration and redress. What's more, disability studies and activism would do well to recognise that the impulse to deny justice to marginalised groups because the conditions of their marginalisation are deemed 'elective' and 'changeable' smacks of neoliberal healthism and is reminiscent of racist, classist, and sexist 'culture of poverty' arguments.[16] To form such alliances, it is also imperative that fat activism and scholarship move away from

---

15 Such a framing might allow for further alliances with groups of other non-normatively bodied individuals, such as transgender and intersex peoples. See Claire (2005).

16 In essence, culture of poverty arguments suggest that cycles of urban poverty, which most directly impact people of colour, are the result, not of structural conditions of inequality, but dysfunctional value systems, passed down from generation to generation, largely by mothers.

the carrot-and-stick goal of defining fatness as necessarily normal and healthy as a means by which to deflect or avoid discrimination (Kirkland 2008). This too is based in neoliberal healthism. Thus, rather than trying to argue for the purity of our actions and therefore the innocence of our fat (LeBesco 2004), we might suggest that an ethos of bodily difference and interdependence is important not just to fat people but for all people, and resist attempts to include our fatness under the banner of normal at the expense of others. Following disability justice, the focus of our activism and the target of our scholarly investigation must therefore shift away from a seeking of inclusion or accommodation, to a dismantling of the social, cultural, and political-economic conditions and structures that create inequality and oppression in the first place.

Queer modes of embodiment – both disabled and fat – expose and resist the illusory nature of normative ideals of autonomy, control, self-determination, and proper citizenship (Garland-Thomson 1997), ideals that I would argue are fundamentally white supremacist, classist, sexist, heterosexist, and cissexist. A critical resistance to and disruption of these categories can make space in our scholarship and our movements for a broad range of experiences that need not be seen as necessarily contradictory: the suffering involved in embodying an outsider status, the seductive pull of normal, the pleasure involved in a moment of transgression, the sadness that results from being excluded, the pain and the messiness of our bodies, the ambivalence and fear we sometimes feel about them, the rage we feel at being denied our humanity, the strength of our desires, and the pleasures our bodies bring to ourselves and others. We might see these experiences, following Wendell (2001), as all contributing to an expanded notion of pride, and moreover, to a notion of justice. And to ensure that our movements are reflective of the broad range of experiences and people within the categories of 'fat' or 'disabled', we must remember that the point of our work, as Haraway (1994 in Shildrick 1996: 13) argues, is not only to trouble the normative and ideological categories 'for the easy frisson of transgression' but rather 'for the hope of livable worlds'.

Acknowledgements

I am grateful to the editors of this volume for their helpful feedback on earlier versions of this chapter and for making space for scholarship on the queerness of fat embodiment.

References

Amphramor, L. 2009. Disability and the anti-obesity offensive. *Disability & Society*, 24(7), 897–909.

Baynton, D.C. 2008. Beyond culture: Deaf studies and the deaf body, in *Open Your Eyes: Deaf Studies Talking*, edited by H.L. Bauman. Minneapolis: The University of Minnesota Press, 293–313.

Bell, C. 2006. Introducing white disability studies: A modest proposal, in *The Disability Studies Reader*, edited by L. Davis. New York: Routledge, 275–282.

Campos, P. 2004. *The Obesity Myth: Why America's Obsession with Weight is Hazardous to Your Health*. New York: Gotham.

Campos, P., Saguy, A., Ernsberger, P., et al. 2006. The epidemiology of overweight and obesity: Public health crisis or moral panic? *International Journal of Epidemiology*, 35, 55–60.

Centers for Disease Control 2009. *U.S. obesity trends: Trends by state 1985–2008*. [Online] Available at: http://www.cdc.gov/obesity/data/trends.html [accessed 17 May 2010].

Chang, V.W. and Christakis, N.A. 2002. Medical modeling of obesity: A transition from action to experience in a 20th century American medical textbook. *Sociology of Health & Illness*, 24(2), 151–177.

Claire, E. 2005. *Toward disability politics of transness*. Politics, Social Change and Justice Conference, New York, May 2005. Available at: http://clags.gc.cuny.edu/downloads/publications/TransProceedings.pdf [accessed 17 May 2010].

Cooper, C. 1997. Can a fat woman call herself disabled? *Disability & Society*, 12(1), 31–41.

Cooper, C. 2010a. *International No Diet Day*. Obesity Timebomb. [Online] Available at: http://obesitytimebomb.blogspot.com/2010/05/international-no-diet-day.html [accessed 17 May 2010].

Cooper, C. 2010b. Fat Studies: Mapping the field. *Sociology Compass*, 4(12), 1020–1034.

Crossley, N. 1995. Merleau-Ponty, the elusive body and carnal Sociology. *Body and Society*, 1(1), 43–63.

Davis, L. 2006. Constructing normalcy: The Bell Curve, the novel and the invention of the disabled body in the Nineteenth Century, in *The Disability Studies Reader*, edited by L. Davis. New York: Routledge, 3–16.

Fine, M. and Asch, A. 1988. Disability beyond stigma: Social interaction, discrimination and activism. *Journal of Social Issues*, 44(1), 3–21.

Foucault, M. 1990. *The History of Sexuality: An Introduction*. New York: Vintage.

Garland-Thomson, R. 1997. *Extraordinary Bodies: Figuring Physical Disability in American Culture and Literature*. New York: Columbia University Press.

Garland-Thomson, R. 2005. Feminist Disability Studies. *Signs: Journal of Women in Culture and Society*, 30(2), 1557–1587.

Hahn, H. 1988. The politics of physical differences: Disability and discrimination. *Journal of Social Issues*, 44(1), 39–47.

Haraway, D. 1994. A game of Cat's Cradle: Science Studies, Feminist theory, Cultural Studies. *Configurations*, 1, 59–71.

Harding, S. and Kirby, M. 2009. *Lessons from the Fat-O-Sphere: Quit Dieting and Declare a Truce with Your Body.* New York: Penguin.

Herndon, A. 2002. Disparate but disabled: Fat embodiment and Disability Studies. *NWSA Journal*, 14(3), 120–137.

Herndon, A.M. 2005. Collateral damage from friendly fire?: Race, nation and class and the 'war against obesity'. *Social Semiotics*, 15, 128–141.

Herrick, C. 2009. Shifting blame/selling health: Corporate social responsibility in the age of obesity. *Sociology of Health & Illness*, 31(1), 51–65.

Hughes, B. 1999. The constitution of impairment: Modernity and the aesthetic of oppression. *Disability & Society*, 14(2), 155–172.

Hughes, B. and Paterson, K. 1997. The social model of disability and the disappearing body: Towards a Sociology of impairment. *Disability & Society*, 12(3), 325–340.

Jutel, A. 2006. The emergence of overweight as a disease entity: Measuring up normality. *Social Science and Medicine*, 63, 2268–2276.

Kelly, J.B. 2002. *Your Sexuality, Your Body, Get Over It!: The Liberatory Ethic of Queer and Disability Theory.* Queer Disability Conference, San Francisco, June 2002. Available at: http://www.disabilityhistory.org/dwa/queer/paper_kelly.html [accessed 17 May 2010].

Kinzel, L. 2008. *Embracing the Morbid.* Two Whole Cakes. [Online] Available at: http://blog.twowholecakes.com/2008/11/embracing-the-morbid/ [accessed 17 May 2010].

Kirkland, A. 2003. Representations of fatness and personhood: Pro-fat advocacy and the limits of the uses of law. *Representations*, 82, 24–51.

Kirkland, A. 2008. Think of the hippopotamus: Rights consciousness in the fat acceptance movement. *Law and Society Review*, 42(2), 397–432.

Kittay, E.P. 2006. Thoughts on the desire for normality, in *Surgically Shaping Children: Technology, Ethics, and the Pursuit of Normality*, edited by E. Parens. Baltimore: Johns Hopkins University Press, 90–112.

Landsman, G. 2009. *Reconstructing Motherhood and Disability in the Age of 'Perfect' Babies.* New York: Routledge.

LeBesco, K. 2004. *Revolting Bodies: The Struggle to Redefine Fat Identity.* Massachusetts: University of Massachusetts Press.

Linton, S. 1998. *Claiming Disability: Knowledge and Identity.* New York: New York University Press.

Mairs, N. 1996. *Waist High in the World: A Life among the Nondisabled.* Boston: Beacon Press.

McRuer, R. 2006. Introduction: Compulsory able-bodiedness and queer/ disabled existence, in *Crip Theory: Cultural Signs of Queerness and Disability*, edited by R. McRuer and M.F. Bérubé. New York: New York University Press, 1–32.

McRuer, R. and Wilkerson, A.L. 2003. Introduction. *GLQ*, 9(1–2), 1–23.

Mingus, M. 2010. *Changing the Framework: Disability Justice – How Our Communities Can Move Beyond Access to Wholeness.* [Online] Available at: http://www. resistinc.org/newsletters/articles/changing-framework-disability-justice [accessed 17 May 2010].

Moll, A. 2007. *The Body Multiple: Ontology in Medical Practice.* Durham: Duke University Press.

Morris, J. 2001. Impairment and disability: Constructing an ethics of care that promotes human rights. *Hypatia*, 16(4), 1–16.

National Association for the Advancement of Fat People. [Online] Available at: http://www.naafaonline.com/ [accessed 17 May 2010].

Nestle, M. 2000. Changing the diet of a nation: Population/regulatory strategies for a developed economy. *Asia Pacific Journal of Clinical Nutrition*, 9(suppl.), S33–S40.

NOLOSE. 2012. *A Response to White Fat Activism from People of Color in the Fat Justice Movement.* [Online] Available at: http://www.nolose.org/activism/ POC.php [accessed 17 May 2010].

O'Toole, C.J. 2004. The sexist inheritance of the Disability Movement, in *Gendering Disability*, edited by B.G. Smith and B. Hutchison. New Brunswick: Rutgers University Press, 294–300.

Oliver, M.J. 1999. The Disability Movement and the professions. *International Journal of Therapy and Rehabilitation*, 6(8), 377–379.

Olkin, R. 1999. *What Psychotherapists Should Know About Disability.* New York: The Guilford Press.

Parens, E. 2006. Introduction: Thinking about surgically shaping children, in *Surgically Shaping Children: Technology, Ethics, and the Pursuit of Normality*, edited by E. Parens. Baltimore: Johns Hopkins University Press, xiii–xxix.

Petersen, A. 2003. Governmentality, critical scholarship, and the Medical Humanities. *Journal of Medical Humanities*, 24, 187–201.

Puhl, R. and Brownell, K.D. 2003. Psychosocial origins of obesity stigma: Toward changing a powerful and pervasive bias'. *Obesity Review*, 4, 213–227.

Rose, N. 2006. *The Politics of Life Itself: Biomedicine, Power and Subjectivity in the Twenty-First Century.* Princeton: Princeton University Press.

Schwartz, H. 1986. *Never Satisfied: A Cultural History of Diets, Fantasies and Fat.* New York: Free Press/Macmillan.

Schwartz, M.B. and Brownell, K.D. 2007. Actions necessary to prevent childhood obesity: Creating the climate for change. *Journal of Law, Medicine & Ethics.* Symposium, 78–89.

Shakespeare, T. 1999. The sexual politics of disabled masculinity. *Sexuality & Disability*, 17(1), 53–65.

Shakespeare, T. and Watson, N. 1996. 'The body line controversy:' A new direction for Disability Studies? *Hull Disability Studies Seminar*. [Online] Available at: http://disability-studies.leeds.ac.uk/files/library/Shakespeare-The-body-line-controversy.pdf [accessed 17 May 2010].

Shakespeare, T. and Watson, N. 2002. The social model of disability. *Research in Social Science and Disability*, 2, 9–28.

Shildrick, M. 1996. Posthumanism and the monstrous body. *Body and Society*, 2(1), 1–15.

Shildrick, M. and Price, J. 1996. Breaking the boundaries of the broken body. *Body and Society*, 2(4), 93–113.

Shuai, T. 2008. *A Different Kind of Fat Rant: People of Color and the Fat Acceptance Movement*. [Online] Available at: http://web.archive.org/web/20100501202 754/http://www.fatshionista.com/cms/index.php?option=com_content&task=view&id=180&Itemid=69 [accessed 17 May 2010].

Solovay, S. 2000. *Tipping the Scales of Justice: Fighting Weight Based Discrimination*. Amherst, New York: Prometheus Books.

Thomas, C. 2004. How is disability understood? An examination of sociological approaches. *Disability & Society*, 19(6), 567–583.

Tremain, S. 2008. Foucault, governmentality, and critical disability theory: An introduction, in *Foucault and the Government of Disability*, edited by S. Tremain. Michigan: University of Michigan Press, 1–26.

Waldschmidt, A. 2008. Who is normal? Who is deviant?: 'Normality' and 'risk' in genetic diagnosis and counseling, in *Foucault and the Government of Disability*, edited by S. Tremain. Michigan: University of Michigan Press, 191–207.

Wann, M. 1999. *Fat! So?: Because You Don't Have to Apologize for Your Size!* California: Ten Speed Press.

Warner, M. 1999. *The Trouble with Normal: Sex, Politics, and the Ethics of Queer Life*. Massachusetts: Harvard University Press.

Wendell, S. 2001. Unhealthy disabled: Treating chronic illnesses as disabilities. *Hypatia*, 16(4), 17–33.

World Health Organization. *Diet and Physical Activity: A Public Health Priority*. [Online] Available at: http://www.who.int/dietphysicalactivity/en/index.html [accessed 17 May 2010].

World Health Organization. *Mental Health: A Call for Action by World Health Ministers*. [Online] Available at: http://www.who.int/mental_health/advocacy/en/Call_for_Action_MoH_Intro.pdf [accessed 17 May 2010].

Chapter 10
Bear Arts Naked: Queer Activism and the Fat Male Body

Scott Beattie

The tactile masculine curves of the hairy bear body stands in stark contrast to the sculpted smooth hard body Adonis prevalent in gay erotica and marketing. The interplay of fat and muscle, hard and soft, gentle and strong opens up wider fields of erotic possibility beyond that of conventionally hard phallic body. In 2012 gay erotic publisher Bruno Gmunder released *Big Love: Sexy Bears in Gay Art*, one of the first commercial collection of bear-themed art, but did this represent a liberation of the gay body from the shackles of the beauty and health industries or merely signify the corporate colonisation of another queer culture?

Bear art suggests queerness in multiple ways, not simply through the homoeroticism of the subject matter. Bear art challenges conventions in the representation of the body, disrupts heterosexual and homosexual norms of masculinity, upsets the depiction of the 'healthy' hard body and blurs the boundaries of techniques representing masculine and feminine through depiction of hardness and softness, muscle and fat. Further, bear art crosses many divides in the artistic field of production, between fine art and commercial art, between professional and amateur, between erotic and pornographic, between multiple online identities, even challenging some assumptions about the consumers and producers of homoerotic art.

The bear body is an emerging site of contestation by conflicting social forces but paradoxically, this takes place on what is often a very ordinary and everyday body. Perhaps this is the key to its disruptive power. It may be that the key challenge of the bear body is to locate these field of disruption not within spectacular contested spaces of gender transgression but within the comfortable bounds of everyday life.

This chapter emerged from a series of interviews with artists who have either identified as bear artists or who have been described as such, seeking an understanding of what bear art was and whether it constituted a form of queer fat activism. While most of the artists denied any overt political agenda, most had little if any connection the bear subculture (many resisting the 'bear art' label altogether), there nevertheless appeared to be a different type of politics emerging, a spatial and discursive politics that opens up fields of possibility rather than confronts dominant hegemonic structures directly. Like the bear body itself, bear art forms a polymorphous field of engagement and that can playfully tease the hierarchies of body fascism.

The research on which this chapter is based began as a series of surveys and interviews with artists whose work could be said to involve 'bear art', although as the process evolved this label became increasingly problematic. A number of artists responded to a short online interview and elaborated their position through further email and social media message conversations. The initial purpose of this research was to explore the politics of bear art, to discern whether there was an activist agenda in challenging fat phobia in art and the media and to see how the art was connected to research which had already been published on bear culture. Further, the questions were designed to probe beyond choice of theme or subject matter to investigate further on issues of technique, to consider how artistic method represents desire, particular in a subject that transgresses social norms of beauty and healthiness. Artists were asked how visual art can convey the sense of touch, what Marks calls a *haptic optics* (2002), in conjuring the alchemy of desire in the interplay of soft and hard forms, a challenge to the 'look but don't touch' hard aloofness of the heroic male ideal.

Most of the artists interview were active online and members of these online art communities such as *DeviantArt* or *Y!Gallery* and also social networks through which they could promote and share artwork. These communities are built around the work itself rather than identity politics or social nexus, so it may be that a sociological, 'subcultural' lens is not the best position from which to understand bear art, rather to look to the artistic and creative networks in which the work circulates. This chapter will explore the idea of *creative counterpublics* as frame of reference, a theory which looks to the relationship between creatives, creative work and their publics (Warner 2002).

Bears, big hairy gay men, are increasingly visible in the mainstream mediascape as well. The bear subculture has its origins in the United states, in bars, zines and small press, but since the 1980s, bears have gradually become more prevalent as an alternative gay body image based on an everyday masculinity (Hennen 2008). The uptake of the bear movement in Asia has challenged both local stereotypes and the 'double stereotype' by through Western gay men can perceive Asian masculinity (Han 2006).

Men who are fat, and even some with average bodies face stereotyping and in the 1990s, in a hedonist gym-centred gay culture, which has been criticised as a form of *body fascism* which renders fat gay men doubly discriminated and outcast (Blotcher 1998), vulnerable to alienation, poor self-esteem, depression and eating disorders and a disconnection from community engagement (Wrench and Knapp 2008). The celebration of the bigger bear body is also in part a response to negative impact of the mainstream culture *obesity crisis* (Gough and Flanders 2009), a health issue which has been described as a moral panic (Monaghan 2006).

It is tempting to see this new visibility of bears as the emergence of a new site of resistance to the hard and slender masculine body image presented by the health and beauty industries as an ideal, even normalised. Could bear culture be understood as a politically engaged subculture contesting the body as a site of conformity? There has been some research concerning the *bear scene* subculture (see for instance Wright 1997, 2001), which has its own verbal and visual cues (calling 'woof' and growling), mores and values, rituals of an outdoorsy bbq culture, and focus on affection and cuddles (Hennen 2008). One surprising factor which emerges from the interview research conducted for this chapter is that 'bear artists' are not necessarily closely connected to bear scene. The artists are not all bears in physical type, they come from a variety of ethnicities across different countries (Hennen 2008 points out how white the bear scene is in the USA) and they are not necessarily identified as gay men, some such as Moonwulf and Yang are in fact women. These interviews have suggested that there is not a simple connection between bear art and the bear subculture and any attempts to describe bear art as an authentic representation of bear culture and values could not be sustained. There are connections, but the relationship between bear aesthetics and identity are more complex.

For the purposes of this chapter the term *bear art* will be used as a collective label but many of the artists expressed reservations about its usefulness, beyond being a marketing label. This is perhaps not surprising as there is no universally accepted definition of what makes a man a bear and even the bear subculture uses a variety of taxonomies including bears, cubs, otters, wolves, even stags (or 'stag hags') who are straight men who like to socialise with bears. Nevertheless, what has been described as Bear Art generally involves masculine men, with visible body hair and are heavier set, 'a man with meat on his bones' (Sepp of Vienna, interview 3/1/12) presenting as a desirable alternative to conventional images of male beauty based on classical heroic ideals.

Bear culture expresses authenticity through naturalness (Hennen 2008) and this idea has resonance in bear art, presenting 'Men's bodies as they actually are' (Steve MacIsaac, interview 12/12/11). This naturalness can be seen as a claim to authentic masculinity but it can also be framed as a resistance the commodification of the body, 'bears are more normal, they are real, real men, not the 'faked gods' of the beauty and health industries. It is an industry just to make money' (Sepp of Vienna, interview 3/1/12). The same claims can be levelled at commercial pornography, Gay pornography is 'almost surreal in its uniformity' of body types (Moonwulf, interview 21/12/11) and bear art presents different bodies as well as different modes of representing intimacy, especially tactile expression through hugs and cuddling.

Some artists were keen to point out that the bear body type, while resisting dominant images, was itself a form of stereotype and they are wary that bear art is becoming a fashion trend like any other (Amir Theamir, interview 12/12/11). Claims of naturalness were also challenged, overall bear art cannot be said to be portraying average men, 'I'd be a lot more impressed if the "range" included average sized (or even small) penises' (Flaming Artist, interview 15/12/11). Not all artists have the ambition of representing normal or even natural bodies. On the contrary, an artist like Logan Kowalsky draw penises which are not realistically sized and feels he has been subject to censorship, not from morals groups but from within gay publishing (Logan Kowalsky, interview 12/12/11).

The issue of fatness gathered a variety of responses from the interviewees. Some artists questioned the conflation of fatness and bear art, seeing them as quite separate categories. For instance Flaming Artist (interview 15/12/11) wondered whether bears belonged in a discussion on queer fatness at all. Are bears fat? Many of the artists interviewed depicted men who were large and massive, but of athletic and muscular build without obvious bellies, see for instance the work of Chris Lopez or Nickie Charles, but nevertheless possess more burly or massive bodies than typical of erotic art.

Fatness (distinct from weight) not an empirical measure, is a socially constructed judgement. Increasingly the use of metrics such as the BMI label more and more men as fat who would not previously have been seen in this way (Evans 2006). The bear body occurs in a range of different weights, but even the most fit and muscular of bears are in peril of facing the negative stereotypes associated with fatness. 'Bears are considered fat. Fat is 'other' in the eyes of the dominant culture and being outside the dominant culture lends one perspective. Men with perspective are usually more interesting. They can see the world more clearly because there is no self-delusion about the world and their place in it. They're also better at sex' (Michael Mitchell, interview 22/12/11).

What Does Bear Art Have to Say?

While appreciating that 'bear art' as a somewhat arbitrary label, there are themes and techniques which many artists share, a conversation in visual language that occurs around the bear body. This section looks at some of the features of this conversation and in the next section Warner's (2002) *counterpublic* concept is used to describe bear art as discursive formation emerging from creative practice rather than as an artefact of subcultural identity politics.

The bear aesthetic emerged from zines and self-published press and these origins cement a connection with an everyday realism (even where it is more a *fantasy* of realism, Hennen 2008) and natural masculinity remains a strong theme for the bear artists interviewed. The different artists use a wide variety of different themes, styles and techniques; from the everyday men of Steve MacIsaac's comics, to others influenced by underground and counterculture art, design work and bar/event promotional art, anthropomorphic or *furry* art, and since the globalisation, Asian styles such as the macho *bara* style of Tagame Gengorah and other mangaka.

Bear art as a technical discourse is also worthy of examination. Beyond the different thematic and ideological codes in the work, there are technical aspects to the representation of big bodies that form a discourse throughout the web of influence and inspirations shared among artists. Across these different styles and genres there are a number of technical intersections resulting from the depiction of the larger, bear body, choices about line weight, colour, shadow and tone that depict the big and hairy body as desirable. Self-proclaimed bear artist Dubon likens the visual language to a code:

> Bear art is a code, as I said, it makes room to alternative aesthetics, Bear art is a different body language. I don't think my bear art rivals the Grecian ideal as the Grecian ideal aims at perfection, aims at being objective and universal. Bear art addresses to the members of the community, doesn't aim at being universal. I don't mean that Grecian ideal "IS" a universal ideal, it was conceived "TO BE" universal. I see the main difference between the two both in the approach and in the audience. (Dubon, interview 10/01/12)

Bear art presents an erotic space of play in which the bear body becomes a field of erotic possibility, where it can be touched. 'I think my favourite bear art will trigger the same sensations as seeing your perfect "type" of guy … certain textures visually lend themselves to feeling, soft, cuddle, scruffy etc. … I've definitely seen images that give me that warm and fuzzy feeling in a major way' (Steve Carrillo, interview 12/12/1). In particular there is a dialectical relationship between hardness and softness, muscle and fat, force and gentleness which is expressed in line weight and light, colour and tone. This play is not overtly political, nor is it meant to represent reality, creation is 'something halfway between reality and fantasy' (Brute by Simon, interview 24/12/11). As such bear art presents its own possibilities which can only be created by art, not words, 'it's a delicate feeling, it's like touching the "Beauty"' (Chris Lopez, interview 13/12/11).

Touching the Bear, a Haptic Visuality

The fatter body presents its own challenges for artists. The idealised *hard body* of fashion, classical art, Western comics and even Manga is self-contained, it follows its own logic of form and construction that can be learnt from anatomical schema. The way that fat bodies occupy space and react to physical forces changes greatly, gravity and inertia shape hard and soft forms, even light falls differently on the skin. Artists move reflexively between depicting what they see (from models or reference) and the anatomy they know from schema such as the Industrial Design method or the Reilly method, a play between inside and outside of bodies. Fatter bodies ask more complicated questions, especially where they are also hairy.

Laura Marks' (2002) concept of *haptic visuality* is useful in describing this play between seeing and touching and the intersubjective relationship by which bodies are produced in discourse. She draws a distinction between optic visuality where the object is contained, described from a distance and haptic visuality which involves a kind of shared embodiment, a different way to represent and experience the body. Haptic visuality embraces the surfaces, is consumed in details and fragments while optic visuality seeks to know the subject from a more objective viewpoint, but these are not mutually exclusive forms of representation. 'The oscillation between the two creates an erotic relationship, a shifting between distance and closeness' (Marks 2002: 13). This itself can have an activist impact, recognising a shift in erotic politics from looking to engaging, seeing the self differently.

Interviewees were asked to discuss the importance of touch in their work. 'Well, if you are really good with certain tools, or tricks, that allow you to give the drawing that "sweaty", "oily" or "moist" feelings, yeah. [Y]ou can allow the viewer to imagine how the drawing would *feel*' (Mark Wulfgar, interview 5/1/12). They reinforced the role of the audience in making this connection with the art (and the artist), 'It is also our imagination in a few lines that would create an impulse of touching and feeling. People are curious, and they need to touch things that they don't feel able to or permitted to touch' (Palanca, interview 22/12/11). Visual art invokes a broad spectrum of senses, 'Smell and hearing are important too. Maybe total sense involvement is what clubbers appreciate in bearparties: socialising, rubbing, smelling, hearing, watching, touching – ok stop, lol' (Amir Theamir, interview 12/12/11).

While it is important not to reify a singular vision of 'bear arts' where none exists, there is clearly a conversation taking place around desire for the bear body in which artist and audiences play off images and technique. This conversation seems to occur parallel to the bear subculture and is not consistently aligned with the social formations, mores and identity practices of that group, nor is membership directly connected (Flaming Artist, interview 15/12/11). However these bodies provide the inspiration for a sexuality alternative to media models of consuming through looking, toward a participatory sexuality expressed through cuddling, mutual touching and play. Artistic technique takes up the challenge of representing this complexity through largely visual codes.

Bear Art as Creative Counterpublic(s)

While the artists creating bear arts seem to enjoy a sense of artistic community, particularly through social networking, this is not determined by nor necessarily connected to the bear scene subculture. While their work resists hegemonic ideas of bodily perfection, many of the artists are reluctant to present their work as political in nature. Rather they foreground aesthetic choice, 'I just create art that I enjoy' (Maleo Lo, interview 22/12/11) and see a need for art to do more than market to a specific subcultural audience (Logan Kowalsky, interview 12/12/11). 'I think creativity is a reaction rather than the beginning. For something to be 'art' I think it has to point out something, at something other than itself' (Grisser, interview 22/12/11).

While the artists do no deny the social connectedness of their art, as a 'measuring stick for culture' (Steve Carrillo, interview 12/12/1), they resist being tied to a subcultural or political movement and are wary of the social taxonomic practices of labelling which occur around gay subcultures and bear cultures specifically (Hennen 2008). 'People tend to put themselves in small boxes and I personally think it's funny to see gay people fighting for their rights and recognition of equality to the world and at the same time arranging their community into smaller ghettoes where others are not always welcome' (Logan Kowalsky, interview 12/12/11).

Aside from some shared values about nature and masculinity it is difficult to make any generalisations about the bears as a political subculture with a set a values or activist goals (Hennen 2005), the scene is organised around aesthetic and bodily practices. Further, Hennen suggests there is a playful and polymorphous eroticism that de-emphasises phallic penetration, where the whole skin becomes a field of erotic play (2005). Manley, Levitt and Mosher (2007) observe there are clusters of meaning involving acceptance, nurturing and physical and emotional intimacy. This emphasis on touch, real or symbolic, is also readily apparent in bear art where the thematic content, as well as the techniques and stylistic conventions produce a haptic visuality. Bear culture and bear art share a set of meanings around the body and masculinity, but these remain fluid and highly contextual.

While it is difficult to align bear art with any authentic subcultural formation, Michael Warner's (2002) formulation of the *counterpublic* concept provides a valuable tool, an alternative way of discussing these sorts of discursive networks. A counterpublic is a relationship between creator, creative work and audience, framed around the concept of the public, both in the social/political sense of the public sphere but also the practical notion of *publication*, Warner provides an alternative way of thinking about creative networks that focuses on the interplay of discourse rather than being concerned with underlying social structures.

A *counterpublic* is emphatically not another term for a subculture or counterculture (although Warner's choice of term does unfortunately contribute to this confusion), but relates both to the publication of media but also the mediated relationship a creator has to 'one's public' through multiple stages of separation, mapped across media networks. An artist, a journalist, a performer, even an academic author engages with their audience and with other creators via a conversation negotiated through the work itself. Warner's theory retains the historical importance of the public while it challenges the liberal idea of universal public sphere, suggesting multiple counterpublics and indeed that 'mainstream public' only represents a narrow set of interests and is just another counterpublic.

Warner's concept differs from previous models such as Nancy Fraser's socio/political counterpublic because the focus is on discourse, and it provides a better framework to understand the role of arts, writers, performers in creating alternative spaces that are flexible, transitory, fragmentary, unstable, but nonetheless important. Each piece of art generates a public as it collects an audience, deployed through time and space, you could speak of a 'bear arts counterpublic' broadly or a specific counterpublic forming around a specific artist's work.

Warner's framework brings bear art away from questions of authenticity and identity politics and sets it free among the complex interplay of discursive networks. It recognises that many different counterpublics challenge the dominance of certain body images in mainstream culture. As a discourse centred theory it also allows us to understand the role of technique and artistic practice in the imagination of alternatives. 'I was brought up on those untouchable gods of gay porn, superhero comics, Manga and they taught me how to draw. When I realised that these were always going to be outside my reach, I had to unlearn it all and find a vocabulary for real bodies and I learned that from other artists whose work turned me on' (Tyr Tapir, interview 7/1/12).

If we recognise that the mainstream body image has an impact on material health, especially for gay men, then, it is important to recognise the hegemonic domain of health and beauty is just a certain form of public (or counterpublic) constituted by the discourse it produces and the resources and techniques which those industries deploy. Bear art challenges this not through hammering home a political message but through imagining a different world of possibility in which different bodies can be desired, and shares its own techniques and visual language to achieve this.

Is Bear Art a Form of Queer Fat Activism?

While Bear Art creates a field of playful images, a contrast to *Mount Olympus* of the heroic male beauty ideals, many of the artists interviewed for this chapter were reluctant to describe their work in terms of political activism. This may be due to the artist's innate suspicion about mixing politics with art (Felshin 1995) or because, on reflection, the questions I asked failed to distinguish between more militant forms of activism and everyday resistance strategies. Further, the disconnect between bear arts and the bear-scene subculture may be another source of anxiety as artists do not want to claim to represent an identity-political authenticity that they do not have.

Nevertheless, artists engage in media discourses that can be both sources of oppression or sites activism, sometimes both. Increasing attention has focussed on media representations of the fat body as the site of hegemonic struggle over the body, Mosher (2001) for instance looks at how mainstream comedy television has engaged with masculinity and the fat male body. By highlighting hypocritical attitudes to fat, Laura Kipnis argues that hard core pornography actually performs a 'social service' by revealing hypocritical attitudes toward fat (Kipnis 1996: 121). Just 'corpulence carries a whole weight as a subversive cultural practice that calls into question received notions about health, beauty and nature. We can recognise fat as a condition not simply aesthetic or medical, but *political*' (LeBesco 2001: 75, emphasis in original).

While acknowledging that creators are cautious about politicising their work, there are at least three ways in which bear art can be understood as a form of queer fat activism, in providing diverse imaginings of the *body*, in presenting an alternative way of expressing *masculinity* based on nurturing touch, and a developing a visual *artistic discourse* around techniques used to represent bodies and space.

The first form of activism acknowledges the harm of negative body image and the importance of establishing new ways of being in one's skin, coming out of the 'second closet' as fat person. Eve Kosofsky Sedgwick emphasises the importance of this dialectic with your own body, that coming out as a fat person is a 'uttering bathetically as a brave declaration that truth which can scarcely in this instance ever have been less than self-evident' that it is 'a way of staking one's claim to insist on, and participate in, a renegotiation of *the representational contract* between one's body and one's world' (Moon and Sedgwick 1990: 255, emphasis in original).

Fatness is a significant issue in the male gay community, where 'body fascism' has been attributed to a form of compound discrimination leading to alienation and outcast status (Blotcher 1998). Giles (1998) observes that the openness with which some gay men feel entitled to belittle and demean fat gay men is similar to the open hatred expressed by homophobes. 'A man thin by straight standards may be considered fat in gay culture' (Mosher 2001: 186). In an empirical study of attitudes, Wrench and Knapp (2008) confirmed the prevalence of image fixation and anti-fat attitudes in the gay male community and the importance of nonverbal communication in conveying these attitudes.

It is important to avoid falling into stereotypes of a singular 'gay community' when discussing body image issues, gay men are still situated in broader social settings (Duncan 2010). Wrench and Knapp (2008) summarised the research into contemporary anti-fat attitudes creating a cluster of stereotypes by which fat people are perceived as indecisive, disorganised, non-industrious, incompetent, self-indulgent, lazy, undisciplined, unfriendly, inactive, possessing poor hygiene, passive, stupid, uncreative and possessing emotional and psychological problems. 'Corpulence studies has developed significant insights into food, gender, sexuality, and the body, specifically in relationship to fat bodies reviled as asexual, out of control, or morally repugnant' (Johnston and Taylor 2008: 945, Braziel 2001). Further, the popularity of the BMI metric in the health industry has meant that fatness becomes a prominent explanation for health problems, one where it is easy to blame the victim and to sell a variety of health solutions based on weight loss products and services (Evans 2006).

Wrench and Knapp (2008: 476) draw a strong connection between image fixation and fat phobia in the male gay community. This emphasises the central role of *imagination* in self-esteem and wellbeing, suggesting the importance of discourse and art in reinforcing or challenging harmful beliefs. The eroticisation of a broader range of body shapes in bear art may lead to greater acceptance among gay men at large, and it can represent an artist's own journey along the path of self-acceptance by breaking the mould of body fascism, 'I had to learn the visual tools by which I could make fatness sexy and through that come to accept my own fat body' (Tyr Tapir, interview 7/1/12). The same could be said for the acceptance of body hair, for both men and women who enjoy the tactile textures of bear art (Yang, interview 22/12/11).

The artists interviewed expressed hope that their art may have a positive effect on the wellbeing of others to have confidence in their bodies (Palanca, interview 22/12/11), that it 'will help men of a different body type understand that, even though they're self-conscious about their shapes and sizes; that there are those of us who truly adore the way that they look, and the way that they are' (Moonwulf, interview 21/12/11). 'Beauty advertising sells a distorted image of ourselves, making us feel different and even ugly. Unconsciously they engage us in a competitive race, becoming anxious if we do not meet the beauty criteria established by society' (Rubo Art, interview 21/12/11). 'The whole "the slimmest you are, the sexier you are" kind of culture that is going on is really damaging our society in various levels. So this could be an ironic way to do a wakeup call' (Mark Wulfgar, interview 5/1/12). Further, those who are do not have bear bodies but who desire them can be affirmed in the legitimacy of their desire, so that they do not 'feel like a weirdo' for loving bigger men (Brute by Simon, interview 24/12/11).

The increasing visibility of the bear body represents one of these kinds of transformations, but as with any field of discourse this is always contested and subject to takeover by hegemonic interests. As bear artists are successful in presenting the bear body as a legitimate site of desire it also becomes commodified, commercialised and risks being co-opted into the body image industries. Bear artist Brute by Simon is concerned that the term 'bear' is distorted and risks losing its meaning especially in relation to bigger bodies, 'nowadays you can find tons of guys who claim to be called "bears" when they've only let their beards grow ... the word "bear" has lost its true essence' (Brute by Simon, interview 24/12/11).

The second form of activism occurs through presenting an alternative form of masculinity that emphasises touch, nurturing and bodily practices of intimacy that express tenderness and emotional warmth. Hugs, cuddles and touching have become core practices of the bear community and important aspects of bear art in the representation of intimacy. Which much of this is coded within a gay sexuality, Kelly and Kane argues that the sexual aspect almost forms an alibi, 'I'm wondering whether this discourse of nurturance has to be presented through a discourse of sex in order to make it OK for men to participate?' (2001: 341).

Hennen suggests that the Bear communities challenge to conventional masculinity draws its power not so much from individual action but from community symbols, 'Bear masculinity must be developed and sustained intersubjectively, within the community itself, an interactive process that is greatly facilitated by the symbol of the bear' (2005: 34). The potency of the bear symbol extends beyond the community itself, as Bear artists share their work in galleries, online and throughout social networks. The iconography Bear has become bigger than can be contained in the bear scene subculture and extends into the broader community as men (and women) explore new ways of expressing masculinity and intimacy.

The third form of activism emerges from the technical aspects of Bear art and the way that the web of influence and inspiration form a discursive fabric between different pieces of art and between different artists. Linework, shade colour and light can contribute to a depiction of fat which is abject or which is desirable. Close textual analysis of written discourse and film are more common, but much less has been written about the techniques and modes of representation of the body in visual art. Much more attention has been paid to the meaning, or the ideological message of a piece of visual art than has been paid to close focus on the techniques themselves.

This is not surprising as there has always been a considerable challenge in providing a written vocabulary and method by which to discuss visual art; to speak about the meaning of line weights and shading, colour and anatomical construction, texture and light. But for artists who are immersed in the counterpublic network of influences and inspiration that comes from being a member of an artistic community, this complex conversation in ingrained in the work itself. I draw hands *this way* because of Tagame Gengorah, *this shadow* is influenced by the way that Chris Lopez plays with light on muscle and *this expression* is borrowed from Steve MacIsaac's clever way of drawing ambiguity.

Can this network of influences and discourse be truly considered a form of activism or is it merely the inward focussed activity of a community of artisans? Designers have struggled with the ethical context of their work, Faud-Luke argues:

> We need visions of beauty – we could call this beauty, "beautiful strangeness", a beauty that is not quite familiar, tinged with newness, ambiguity and intrigue, which appeals to our innate sense of curiosity … beauty that is more than skin deep, beauty that is envisioned by society, because the current version of beauty is largely ordained by big-business and governments. We need a beauty that serves in all society, healing society's divides. (2012: 188)

In each of these three strategies bear art activism contributes to a different way of seeing, a break from the body fascism of smooth young hard bodies. Desire is a complex phenomenon and it would be unlikely that a single artistic image (from bear art or any discourse) would entirely shift an individual's sexual destiny, but conversely if certain body types are not visible in the media landscape it is that much harder for these to find their way *on the menu* of desire.

Bear artists provide an alternative, a counterpublic space to desire and to know that you are capable of being desired. Bear artists build a shared space a tactile imaginary terrain where creative forces are catalysed, opening the field of playful possibilities for erotic in hard and soft, muscle and fat, hair and skin, strength and gentleness. Direct activist politics around fatness and acceptance, along with the subversion of hegemonic images are important (Whitesel 2007) but there also remains room for playful touching, expanding the range of possibilities through erotic art. Through social networking and various online and offline distribution possibilities, these counterpublics make a credible force for change that need not be constrained by essentialist identities or subcultural formations, nor have any need to be connected to authentic politics of an activist group or culture. Bear arts can be understood as an aesthetic and discursive force rather than a social and political one without diluting its power to effect change.

References

Blotcher, J. 1998. Justify my love handles: How the queer community trims the fat, in *Looking Queer: Body Image and Identity in Lesbian, Bisexual, Gay and Transgender Communities*, edited by D. Atkins. New York: Harrington Park Press, 359–366.

Braziel, J.E. 2001. Sex and fat chics: Deterritorializing the fat female body, in *Bodies Out of Bounds: Fatness and Transgression*, edited by J.E. Braziel and K. LeBesco. Berkeley: University of California Press, 231–256.

Duncan, D. 2010. Embodying the gay self: Body Image, reflexivity and embodied identity. *Health Sociology Review*, 19(4), 437–350.

Evans, B. 2006. 'Gluttony or sloth': Critical geographies of bodies and morality in (anti)obesity policy. *Area*, 38(3), 259–267.

Faud-Luke, A. 2012. *Design Activism: Beautiful Strangeness for a Sustainable World*. Hoboken: Earthscan.

Felshin, N. 1995. *But is it Art? The Spirit of Art Activism*. Seattle: Bay Press.

Giles, P. 1998. A matter of size, in *Looking Queer: Body Image and Identity in Lesbian, Bisexual, Gay and Transgender Communities*, edited by D Atkins, New York: Harrington Park Press, 355–357.

Gough, B. and Flanders, G. 2009. Celebrating 'obese' bodies: Gay 'Bears' talk about weight, body image and health. *International Journal of Mens' Health*, 8(3), 235–253.

Han, A. 2006. 'I think you're the smartest race I've ever met': Racialised Economies of queer male desire. *Australian Critical Race and White Studies E-journal*, 2(2), 1–14.

Hennen, P. 2005. Bear bodies, Bear masculinity: Recuperation, resistance or retreat? *Gender and Society*, 19(1), 25–43.

Hennen, P. 2008. *Faeries, Bears and Leathermen: Men in Community Queering the Masculine*. Chicago: University of Chicago Press.

Johnston, J. and Taylor, J. 2008. Feminist consumerism and fat activists: A comparative study of grassroots activism and the Dove Real Beauty Campaign. *Signs*, 33(4), 941–966.

Kelly, E.A. and Kane K. 2001. In Goldilocks's footsteps: Exploring the discursive construction of gay sexuality in Bear magazines, in *The Bear Book II*, edited by LK Wright. New York: Harrington, 327–350.

Kipnis, L. 1996. *Bound and Gagged: Pornography and the Politics of Fantasy in America*. New York: Grove.

LeBesco, K. 2001. Queering fat bodies/politics, in *Bodies out of Bounds: Fatness and Transgression*, edited by J.E. Braziel and K. LeBesco. Berkeley: University of California Press, 74–90.

Manly, E., Levitt, H. and Mosher, C. 2007. Understanding the Bear Movement in gay male culture. *Journal of Homosexuality*, 53(4), 89–112.

Marks, L.U. 2002. *Touch: Sensuous Theory and Multisensory Media.* Minneapolis: University of Minnesota Press.

Monaghan, L.F. 2006. Weighty words: Expanding and embodying the accounts framework. *Social Theory and Health*, 4, 128–167.

Moon, M. and Sedgwick, E.K. 1990. Divinity: A dossier a performance piece a little understood emotion. *Discourse*, 13(1), 12–39.

Mosher, J. 2001. Setting free the Bears: Refiguring fat men on television, in *Bodies out of Bounds: Fatness and Transgression*, edited by J.E. Braziel and K. LeBesco. Berkeley: University of California Press, 166–196.

Warner, M. 2002. *Publics and Counterpublics.* New York: Zone Books.

Whitesel, J. 2007. Fatvertising: Reconfiguring fat gay men in cyberspace. *Limina: A Journal of Historical and Cultural Studies*, 13, 92–102. Available at: http://www.limina.arts.uwa.edu.au/__data/page/59120/Whitesel.pdf [accessed 7 June 2013].

Wrench, J.S. and Knapp, J.S. 2008. The effects of body image perceptions and sociocommunicative orientations on self-esteem, depression, and identification and involvement in the gay community. *Journal of Homosexuality*, 55(3), 471–501.

Wright, L. 1997. *The Bear Book: Readings in the History and Evolution of a Gay Male Subculture.* New York: Harrington Park Press.

Wright, L. 2001. *The Bear Book II: Further Readings in the History and Evolution of a Gay Male Subculture.* New York: Harrington Park Press.

Thanks to the artists who participated in this project, their online galleries provide further examples of the work in this field.

Amir Theamir http://www.flickr.com/theamir, http://amirtheamir.blogspot.com
Brute by Simon Http://www.brutebysimon.com
Chris Lopez http://www.lopezgallery.com
Dubon http://bear-art.dubon.eu
Flaming Artist http://www.flamingartist.com
Grisser http://yaoi.y-gallery.net/user/grisser, http://www.furaffinity.net/user/grisser
Logan Kowalsky http://www.loganporncomics.org/
Mark Wulfgar http://yaoi.y-gallery.net/user/markwulfgar/
Mauleo Lo http://mauleo-comic.blogspot.com
Michael Mitchell http://www.hjmag.com/handjobseroticartpage.html
Moonwulf http://yaoi.y-gallery.net/user/moonwulf/
Palanca http://www.palancafeet.blogspot.com
Rubo Art http://www.ruboart.blogspot.com
Sepp of Vienna http://www.sepp-of-vienna.at
Steve Carrillo http://m3llo.deviantart.com/

Steve MacIsaac http://www.stevemacisaac.com
Tyr Tapir http://Www.tyrtapir.blogspot.com
Yang http://yaoi.y-gallery.net/user/yang, http://yang.deviantart.com

Chapter 11
Fashion's 'Forgotten Woman': How Fat Bodies Queer Fashion and Consumption

Margitte Kristjansson

Although many studies refute a simple correlation between weight gain and overeating, ... American culture still sees fat only in terms of self-indulgence. (Hartley 2001: 66)

Conditioned to lose control at the mere sight of desirable products, we can master our desires only by creating rigid defences against them. The slender body codes the tantalising ideal of the well-managed self in which all is kept in order despite the contradictions of consumer culture; the fat body is thus seen 'as an extreme capacity to capitulate to desire', an idea that is rooted in the consumer-culture construction of desire as overwhelming and overtaking the self (Bordo 1993: 201).

Fat people, so the cultural logic goes, are consumers who *over*-consume: the material evidence of their corpulence is 'proof' of this. Fat women in particular experience a double-bind in this regard: while their fatness represents an inability to exercise proper consumptive control, their status as *women* renders their desire for consumption taboo and potentially dangerous. In *Unbearable Weight* (1993), Susan Bordo asserts that for women, the desire to eat – voraciously or otherwise – is conflated with inappropriate sexual desire. The consuming woman as metaphor, she argues, is about the fear that women will literally 'consume the body and soul of the male' and thus their appetites 'must be curtailed and controlled' (117). In other words, the fat woman is figured as deviant not only for her 'obvious' overconsumption, but for the fact that she consumes at all. Fat people more generally, with their out-of-control bodies and apparent inability to resist the temptations of consumer culture, are not commonly understood as particularly sophisticated consumers. As a result, fat-specific consumption practices are currently under-theorised. What is there to study, after all, if the fat consumer will eat or buy anything?

Through an analysis of fat fashion, I will attempt to explore some of the ways that the fat female body both exposes the cultural dimensions of fat consumption practices and is also capable of queering those consumption practices. I use 'queering' here to point to an intentional subversion of cultural norms about consumption – that is who is allowed to consume and how much and in what ways – but, as fat studies scholar Kathleen LeBesco deftly explores in her chapter on queerness and fat in *Revolting Bodies?* (2004), the fat female body can be read as 'queer' in several respects, an interesting consideration I will return to later. An article published in *The New York Times* in 1969 – 'The Forgotten Woman in the "Skinny Revolution"' – is an example of early explorations into fat consumption practices and operates as a catalyst here to consider the ways in which fat women have consumed fashion since the 1960s. This chapter is buoyed by historical examples, but also uses work on fat female subjectivity by Michael Moon and Eve Sedgwick, Kathleen LeBesco, Samantha Murray, and others to situate this discussion at the intersections of issues about race, gender, class and sexuality *as well as* size in order to explore the consumption of fat fashion as an act that queers what we believe to be true about fat bodies and possibly consumption itself.

Taste, Cultural Capital and the Fat Consumer

In his extensive scholarship on consumption practices and social class, Pierre Bourdieu emphasises the importance of cultural capital, 'anything that a society recognises as meaningful, valuable, or estimable [that] can be cultivated for social profit, exchanged for other forms of power, and subject to the range of strategies commonly associated with economic manoeuvring' (Gerber and Quinn 2008: 5). That is, while economic capital remains the central mode of power in society, a recognition of the influence of *cultural* capital is necessary to any understanding of how power is negotiated in and through society. Bourdieu argues that taste – that is, stylised and valorised preferences within consumption practices – operates as a mechanism for distinguishing between those with varying amounts and types of cultural capital. These 'manifested preferences' are 'the practical affirmation of an inevitable difference ... asserted purely negatively, by the refusal of other tastes' (Bourdieu 1984: 56). In other words, one of the ways in which we distinguish ourselves from cultural and social 'others' is through our taste as well as through *dis*taste, disgust, and aesthetic intolerance. Similarly, Deborah Lupton further examines how taste is used to mask cultural privilege. According to Lupton, 'taste is both an aesthetic and a moral category ... a way of subtly identifying and separating 'refined' individuals from the lower, 'vulgar' classes. Good taste is something that is *acquired through acculturation* into a certain subculture rather than being explicitly taught' (1996: 95, emphasis added). Similarly, Gerber and Quinn argue that preferences in consumption make the effects of social and cultural privilege 'appear to be the result of individual refinement rather than social structure and the different kinds of power which animate it' (2008: 5).

As fat studies scholars have maintained, fat bodies are particularly disadvantaged in terms of cultural capital (Gerber and Quinn 2008, LeBesco 2004). In a culture that values slimness over corpulence as not only more beautiful or desirable but also more moral and good, fatness has a negative effect on one's cultural capital and, subsequently, one's ability to acquire other types of capital. Importantly, Bourdieu argues that one of the most significant aspects of cultural capital is its embeddedness within the body: 'the body is the most indisputable materialisation of class tastes' (1984: 190). While 'one's taste might be expressed through the relatively transitory choices made in commodity consumption – how one dresses, the style in which one's house is decorated – [it] is represented and reproduced in a far more permanent way through embodiment' (Lupton 1996: 95). The thin body is read as moral/good/controlled/refined. This is because, in part, the thin body is never regarded as a 'natural' body. As Bourdieu asserts, 'the legitimate use of the body is spontaneously perceived as an index of moral uprightness, so that its opposite, a 'natural' body, is seen as an index of *laisser-aller* ('letting oneself go'), a culpable surrender to facility' (1984: 193). The thin body, for most people, is only attainable through rigorous effort, requiring time and money. And yet, as Gerber and Quinn assert, 'efforts at controlling body size … rarely result in the desired bodily capital': this has the effect of 'guaranteeing the rarity of 'ideal weight' and thus its value' as a kind of cultural capital (2008: 6).

Read any number of news pieces on the 'obesity epidemic' and it is clear that fat people have become a scapegoat of sorts for a lot of the Western world's worst qualities. More often than not, they are imagined as one large homogenous group that exemplify all that is 'wrong' with Western culture: they drive around in gas-guzzling SUVs, watch endless hours of TV on expensive plasma screens, and eat mindlessly out of fast food containers, all while remaining miraculously ignorant of basic health principles and the environmental impact of their selfish consumption practices. As a culture, we seem to be unable to disconnect the metaphor of fatness from its reality. Fat folks, just like their thin or 'average' sized counterparts, consume food (healthy and unhealthy), buy cars (hybrids and gas-guzzlers alike), purchase homes, and consume many other necessary (and not-so-necessary) products. On the other hand, as cultural outsiders with sometimes-limited access to the capital required to engage in normative consumption practices, many fat people are required to consume differently. Importantly, this point is especially true with regard to the consumption of fashion. Due to historically unequal access to clothing in fat sizes, the consumption of fat fashion has happened in very different ways than the consumption of what is often referred to as 'straight-sized' fashion.

The late nineteenth and early twentieth centuries in the United States saw the birth of the department store and the growth of the 'ready-to-wear' fashion industry (Leach 1984). A history of ready-to-wear fashion in America made specifically for fat women can be traced to Lithuanian immigrant Lena Bryant, who, in the 1920s, turned her maternity-wear line into a clothing company for 'stout' women, the first of its kind (Clifford 2010). Today, Lane Bryant is one of the most prominent and prolific plus-size retailers in the country. The plus-size market has seen growth above and beyond the fashion industry at large, and events such as Full Figured Fashion Week in New York City are gaining in popularity (ibid.). Online, a transnational movement of fat fashion bloggers has sparked a mini-frenzy of media attention and body-positive activism (Cochran 2010). 'If the personal is political', writes social commentator Erin Keating, 'than being able to find clothes that fit and make you feel good is a political plus' (quoted in LeBesco 2004: 72). In an industry where the fat fashionista has been called the 'forgotten woman' – a plus-size store with this name existed in New York in the 1980s – the possibilities for her today seem much improved. However, as many fat fashion bloggers are quick to point out, the physical and economic accessibility of fashionable clothing for fat women is still a major issue, and it continues to bring many young and dissatisfied people into the fold of fat- and body-positive activism. Fat fashion, asserts fat studies scholar Kathleen LeBesco, has the capacity to be 'revolutionary': when fat women 'disdain "blending in" in favour of cobbling together a look from the scattered resources available and becoming more brave about appearing in ways that defy the "tasteful" intentions of the commodities of corpulence' they subvert cultural norms about what it means to be fat (2004: 73). Unequal access to fat-sized fashion is a well-documented and long-term phenomenon (Klemesrud 1969, Riggs 1983, Feuer 1999, Adam 2001, LeBesco 2004, Kinzel 2012). Even now, after several decades of fat-positive activism and consumer interest fuelling the creation of more fat fashion, clothing in larger sizes is not nearly as accessible as 'straight-sized' clothing, in terms of quantity as well as quality. As such, today's fa(t)shionistas have developed their own ways to engage with fashion when the industry refuses to recognise them as viable customers. This has manifested itself in hundreds of fatshion blogs, community-building events such as fat-only clothing swaps, online fatshion-centred communities and forums, independent fat-positive fashion shows, and the creation of zines and even documentaries cataloguing the efforts of fat women to render their bodies visible via the fashion that they consume. And while today's fatshion scene is very focused on the present, I would like to point to an important historical moment, while fat-positive activism was still in its infancy, to highlight and analyse the ways in which fat bodies not only queer normative consumption of fashion, but are, in and of themselves, queer.

The 'Forgotten Woman' in 1969

'The Forgotten Woman in the "Skinny Revolution"' appeared in the 'Food Fashions Family Furnishings' section on page 58 of *The New York Times* on Monday, December 1, 1969. It occupies just under half the page, and underneath it are articles about a curmudgeonly English chef and his large, American-style New York City banquet, a profile on Broadway actress-turned-marine biologist Sylvia Short and her family, and the grand opening of a specialty chocolate shop at Bloomingdale's. On the bottom left hand corner is an advertisement for Faberge Cologne (with a new bottle design 'she'll covet almost as much as the fragrance itself') also exclusive to Bloomingdale's. To the contemporary reader, the placement of a story about fat fashion and issues of accessibility might seem odd nestled atop fluff pieces about gourmet chocolate and socialite banquets. The piece on Sylvia Short, a woman who left show business to pursue her doctorate, also seems out of place here. However, when it is revealed that Short chose to quit her career as an actress because day-care costs became too expensive (her husband, also an actor, chose to stay on Broadway and later won a Tony for his efforts), the organisation of these articles and their placement under the decidedly feminine catchall 'Food Fashions Family Furnishings' become a little clearer.

Klemesrud covered a myriad of topics in her 19 years at the paper, including articles about the accessibility of jobs in the fashion industry for African-Americans, the women's liberation movement and its various influences on everyday life, and a small handful of articles about the intersections of fashion, fat, and food. In one such article from 1975 titled 'The Woman Who Isn't Slim Desires High Fashion, Too' Klemesrud quotes a fat woman who suspects that, 'because of women's lib, we're going to have a lot more big women': 'women are tired of the façade and the false eyelashes, and finally we're saying "we're just going to be ourselves"' (45). Fashion in *The New York Times*, at least in the late 60s and 70s, is here configured as an inherently feminine interest. (Other female-gendered interests include of course 'food, family, [and] furnishings'.) This is hardly surprising, given that shopping has historically been coded as a female – or at least feminine – activity (Leach 1984, Abelson 1989, Miller 1998). In general, the interventions made in Klemesrud's articles seem to be at least subtly influenced – if not intentionally so – by the women's liberation movement and the increasing demands from women for more access and more options.

In a similar vein, 'The Forgotten Woman' tells the stories of eight fat women – all wealthy, many of them famous – and their various difficulties finding clothes that fit well and are fashionable. Klemesrud blames the 'skinny revolution' – ostensibly a trend in fashion attributed to famously slender supermodel Twiggy – for these difficulties. 'I think it's the worst thing that's ever happened to heavy women. There is hardly a dress made over size 14', laments Totie Fields, the unapologetically fat comedian. Along with Fields, the women profiled by Klemesrud are New York restaurateur Elaine Kaufman, opera singer Eileen Farrell, Cass Elliot of popular vocal group The Mamas and the Papas, President of the UN General Assembly Angie Brooks of Liberia, owner of the New York Mets Mrs Charles Shipman Payson, the New Jersey governor's wife Mrs Richard J. Hughes, and popular singer Kate Smith. For almost every woman featured, the solution to the problem of accessibility is to have her clothes made for her, or, in the case of Angie Brooks, to make them herself. Fields is quoted as saying she spends as much as $100,000 a year (over $500,000 in 2012 dollars) on her entirely custom-made wardrobe. This is of course only an option, Klemesrud admits, for 'women of means' such as those listed above.

An interesting pattern appears as Klemesrud continues her story: 'Miss Fields, whose weakness is rye bread' is followed by 'Miss Smith, who has gone from 255 pounds to 185 pounds' which is followed by 'Mrs Charles Shipman, known for her fondness for hot dogs, peanuts, ice cream, chocolate bars, and Cokes' which is followed by 'Mrs Hughes, who received nationwide publicity when she dieted and went from 230 to 150 pounds. (She has since gained back 23 of them)'. Although the topic at hand is clothing, the things Klemesrud finds worth noting about these women are inextricably linked to culturally ingrained assumptions about fat women (that they overeat) and their habits (that they are trying to lose weight). Many of the women offered up this information on their own: 'eight years ago I quit smoking and gained 30 pounds. But that's no excuse', confesses Shipman, 'I've always been big'. Most of these women, Klemesrud concludes, fall under one of two categories: those who celebrate their size by wearing loud and/or revealing clothing, and those who use clothing to hide or minimise their corpulence. The opera diva Eileen Farrell is pictured in the top left of the article, wearing a no-nonsense dark suit and helping herself to what looks like pasta. The caption reads, 'Eileen Farrell, the soprano, who frequently goes on diets, prefers to wear dark-coloured fashions'. Kate Smith, likewise, 'always wear[s] sleeves' to hide her 'ham'-like upper arms. Elaine Kauffman, on the other hand, chooses loud prints while Cass Elliot and Mrs Richard J. Hughes dare to wear pants, apparently a fashion don't for fat women in the late 60s. Totie Fields 'break[s] all the rules': 'ruffles, ostrich feathers, fox coats. You look fat in fox anyway, so if you start fat, you only look a little bit fatter'.

It seems easy, then, to assume that Klemesrud is correct in her assertion about these two types of fat women, but a closer reading of the text troubles this simple conception of fat female identities as either celebratory and self-accepting or unhappy and self-hating.

Totie Fields, who for all intents and purposes embodies the ultimate 'if you've got it, flaunt it' fat woman, explains her desire to create a plus-size fashion line inspired by her own striking style. The sizes, she says, would be marked 'in the tiny sizes of 3, 5 and 7' (typically plus-sizes today are sizes 14+). 'Mentally, it will make us feel better', she says. Perhaps in the article it is assumed that the experience of being fat is universally negative, but this statement, made without any comment by Klemesrud, seems to betray the conception of Fields as a revolutionary who loves her body. Similarly, the restaurateur Elaine Kaufman, who says of her fashion sense 'the bolder the better', admits to an ambivalence about her body that isn't fully drawn out by Klemesrud: 'I never quite think of myself as 'big' but I know I must be because my dresses take up a lot of fabric'. And then, when telling the story of how a 'very beautiful – but very unhappy' fashion model asked her why she refused to lose weight, Kaufman retorts, 'I am involved in the mind, and that's all that matters'. For all the work these women seem to be doing to advance some sort of ideology of 'body acceptance' or celebration of the fat female form, they don't seem particularly happy with their size (Fields) or even aware of themselves as being *connected* to their fat bodies (Kaufman).

Consumption and Fat Female Subjectivity

The inclusion of only wealthy – and almost entirely white – women in this article is not incredibly surprising, but is still worth noting. On the one hand, wealthy fat women have access to personal tailors and clothes custom-made by designers and costumers to a much larger degree than women who do not have the same economic and cultural capital. On the other hand, as LeBesco points out, fat bodies in America are threatening inasmuch as they suggest not only 'downward mobility' but 'provoke racial anxieties in the West because of their imagined resemblance to those of maligned ethnic and racial Others; fatness haunts as the spectre of disintegrating physical privilege' (2004: 56). More recently, Amy Erdman Farrell has elaborated on the links between colonialist discourses around non-white bodies, contemporary racism, and the cultural distaste for fat (2011). Presenting the fat woman as a worthy consumer of fashion is then more 'palatable' if the woman we are confronted with is as un-Other as possible. A woman who, although fat, has the taste and distinction of one who possesses great social and cultural capital: '… the spaces defined by preferences in food, clothing or cosmetics are organised according to the same fundamental structure, that of the social space determined by volume and composition of capital' (Bourdieu 1984: 208). After all, how threatening to the status quo can 'Mrs Charles Shipman' be, as a wealthy white woman with a husband to boot? In other words, the subversive potential of the article is tempered by its focus on subjects who, beyond their desire to disrupt fashion norms, have a vested interest in maintaining the status quo. The inclusion of the more body-positive and feminist-leaning Fields, along with Angie Brooks, a black woman and Liberian political leader, is perhaps reflective of the influence of the Civil Rights and Women's Liberation movements of the 1960s.

It could be argued that a relatively positive article about fat women, appearing in such a widely read and well-regarded paper, is reflective of a cultural shift perhaps inspired by women's lib. Of course there are tensions when naming the move to demand increased access to fashionable clothing as 'liberatory' or even 'feminist'. Danae Clark, in her 1991 essay 'Commodity Lesbianism', warns of the kind of commodification that looks like acceptance or even empowerment but is actually about a business's bottom line: the capitalist is happy to welcome queer folk as 'consuming subjects' but remains unwilling to acknowledge them as 'social subjects' (192). Similar arguments can be made for the fat consumer. As LeBesco explains, the demand for increased access to fashionable clothing for fat women often requires insisting that fat women want to be beautiful, too, and reinforces a particular kind of female subjectivity that, in a capitalist society, can only be accessed through consumption. In this way, 'the objectification against which feminists have been fighting for decades becomes the new dream state of the fat woman consumer' (2004: 68). In 1969, when women's lib found many thin women choosing to buck fashion trends and the cultural imperatives to present themselves in traditionally 'beautiful' ways, the fat woman was fighting to be recognised as someone worthy of these things in the first place. This is problematic, yes, but not a simple reproduction of patriarchy and other cultural norms as some might argue, a point I will return to later. Nevertheless, the 'fat woman in a clothing store', Sedgwick asserts, 'lights up a pinball machine of economic, gender, and racial meanings' (2001: 294) and offers interesting ways to think about female subjectivity through consumption. The fat woman shopping is plagued by a 'primal denial', ... the mostly unspoken sentence ... 'there's nothing here for you to spend your money on' (ibid.). Historical analyses of the female shopper have already explicated a complex relationship between the development of female political subjectivity and shopping since the beginnings of modern consumer culture (Leach 1984, Rappaport 2000) – what does this mean, then, for the fat woman who for so long has had little or nothing to buy?

> This is a dream I had a couple of years ago. I was shopping for clothes for myself at a store that was nominally Bloomingdale's. I was dubious about whether they would have any clothes that would be big enough for me, but a saleswoman said they did, adding that rather than being marked by size numbers, each size-group of clothes was gathered under a graphic symbol: over here, she said were the clothes that would fit me. "Over here" referred to a cluster of luscious-looking clothes, hung on a rack between two curtained dressing rooms. The graphic

symbol that surmounted them was a pink triangle. I woke up extremely cheerful. (Moon and Sedgwick 2001: 292)

In their musings on the 'glass closet', Michael Moon and Eve Sedgwick draw parallels between non-normative (queer?) bodies and non-normative (queer) sexualities. 'Closet of sexuality. Closet of size. … What kind of secret can the body of a fat woman keep?' asks Moon (305). After all, he asserts, everyone who sees a fat woman believes 'they know something about her that she doesn't herself know' much in the way that gay people have reported coming out to friends and family members who, instead of being surprised, respond with relief that they can publicly acknowledge what they already believed to be true (ibid.). But, Sedgwick adds, there is more to the 'closet' as it functions in a fat woman's life, whether literally as a container for clothes that do not exist or as a place to keep a secret that everyone already knows:

There *is* a process of *coming out as a fat woman*. [It] involves … risk [and] making clear to the people around one that their cultural meanings will be, and will be heard as, assaultive and diminishing to the degree that they are not fat-affirmative. [It] is a way of speaking one's claim to insist on, and participate actively in, a renegotiation of *the representational contract* between one's body and one's world. (306)

In her chapter on 'The Queerness of Fat', LeBesco explores the many parallels between fatness and queerness, including the above-mentioned concern with 'coming out', early scientific understandings of fat and queer bodies as the product of either environmental factors or genetics ('cause-seeking rhetoric'), and an understanding of both fat and queer sexuality as deviant (2001: 85–88). In fact, fat and queer author Hanne Blank maintains that 'because fat people are not supposed to be sexy or sexual, any sex involving a fat person is by definition "queer", no matter what the genders of any of the partners involved' (quoted in LeBesco 2001: 89).

Shortly after discussing the 'coming out' process for fat women, Moon and Sedgwick go on to briefly summarise the emerging 'fat liberation movement' which, at least in 1993, was attempting the 'liberatory moment of ontologic *di*slinkage' (307), questioning and subverting what was believed to be true of fat bodies from a scientific standpoint. Klemesrud's article comes at an interesting time, then, as 1969 marks the genesis of this movement. Just nine months after 'The Forgotten Woman', *The New York Times* published 'There Are a Lot of People Willing to Believe Fat is Beautiful' an article by Klemesrud about the emergence of NAAFA (then the National Association to Aid Fat Americans, today the National Association to Advance Fat Acceptance). William Fabrey, the founder, is here positioned as a fat admirer, a thin person who prefers fat women as sexual partners. It is not coincidental that then, as is often the case today, a fat woman's worth is asserted based on her ability to appeal to heterosexual men as an object of desire. Even the article itself is couched in a way that problematically ties the fat woman's subjectivity with the male gaze's objectification of her body. However, in 'Averting the Male Gaze: Visual Pleasure and Images of Fat Women' (1999), Jane Feuer argues that 'we need to distinguish among issues involving the male gaze, those involving norms of beauty culture at a given time, and those involving body size per se ... It is only by approximating other norms of beauty culture and thus evoking a male gaze that fat women today can gain access to representation in a form that does not code them as repellent' (185). In a world where fat women experience what Feuer terms 'visual oppression' – a complete lack of positive representation in visual media – 'representation as objects of visual pleasure is progressive' (198). This is especially true, she adds, when the images are being consumed by a female/lesbian spectator.

Still, it could be argued that the subversive potential of fat women's participation in fashion is necessarily mitigated by heteronormative expectations of femininity. How is a woman wearing a fancy dress, for example, non-normative in any way? However, the fat woman is always already figured as *outside of* these expectations – so when she chooses to dress 'femme', she is faced with entirely different readings of her femininity (and thus, her status as an object of desire) by others. 'The fat woman is a masquerade of femininity', Feuer asserts, 'as the figure of Divine well parodies' (186). Rather than painstakingly attempting to reproduce femininity, many fat women are 'playing at' the feminine in ways that feel empowering to them *outside of* patriarchal beauty norms. This understanding of fat femme as subversive performance must, of course, be attentive to intentionality. Even still, heteronormative expectations of femininity are such that fat women can *never fully meet them* – whether now or in 1969 – thus rendering the fat woman's participation in fashion necessarily different.

While it is clear that Klemesrud's 'Forgotten Woman' has many desires, her sexuality is generally avoided in favour of highlighting a lust for fashion and, problematically, food. Only one woman, Mrs. Hughes, is represented as a sexual subject, and this characterisation is itself a bit of a stretch: 'my mother told me I looked terrible in pants, but my husband said I looked great' she says. The reason she is comfortable breaking this fashion 'rule', at least according to her, is because of the validation provided by her husband that she is attractive and thus desirable. This is the only mention of fat women and sexuality, and yet the article is littered with language that is often used when describing sexual desire: Totie Fields is rendered 'weak', some of the women 'flaunt' what they've 'got', Mrs Charles Shipman has a 'fondness', and Cass Elliot is caught 'mooning over'. These words do not describe the desire these women have for *other bodies*, but for food they should not be eating, and rule-breaking outfits they should not be wearing. This erasure of fat women as sexual subjects (or instead the depiction of fat women as sexual beings who desire food) might not be surprising to Petra Kuppers, whose essay about fat, feminist performance explores how the same binaries that govern how we conceptualise sexuality also govern how we perceive the consumption of food, which perhaps allows for an understanding of food *as* desirable, even sexually gratifying (2001). Bordo's assertion, that we conflate a woman's desire to eat with sexual desire, and that the slender body represents proper restraint with regard to both sex and food, is also particularly salient here (1993). Moon and Sedgwick find similar parallels in the films of John Waters and his muse, fat drag queen Divine. Klemesrud's 'Forgotten Woman' lives a life of excess: too much food, too much fabric, and a body that takes up too much space. Obscuring her sexual subjectivity in food talk could be read as an attempt to render the subversive excessiveness of her body 'safe'. Dieting is the only 'proof' a fat woman has that she is at least trying to take 'control' of her body (and thus her sexuality): it is not surprising, then, that Klemesrud focuses so much attention on the eating patterns of these women.

Body 'Language'

Language, as a tool that can be used to reinforce or reinscribe power relations, is especially important when we consider the body and how we talk about it. Many social justice movements have taken to 'reclaiming' the words that have been used to disempower marginalised groups in the past: similarly, the fat-positive movement from the very beginning has privileged 'fat' over other words to describe fat bodies. Despite this, euphemisms for fat continue to be used more often than not. In 'The Forgotten Woman', Klemesrud (or the fat women themselves) use the following descriptors: 'larger women', 'heavy women', 'her "football player figure"', 'stout women', 'big', and 'sizeable'. Notably, the only woman who calls herself fat is Totie Fields, and the only other occurrence of the word is used by Klemesrud to describe Fields's line of clothing for 'fat women'; it is certainly possible that Klemesrud was either asked by Fields to word it this way, or only felt comfortable using the word after Fields herself used it.

These euphemisms are used to make fat women feel better, so as not to risk offending them by using a word that has often been used to belittle or hurt them. But the choice certainly seems puzzling: like the glass closet, what does calling a fat woman 'heavy' or 'stout' *really* do? It certainly cannot hide the fact that she is fat. But the pervasive use of euphemisms for fat bodies sheds some light on why many fat women, like Sedgwick, feel the need to 'come out as fat': not only is it a declaration of one's commitment to the resignification of the fat body, but it is the refusal to metaphorically hide one's body behind words like 'voluptuous' or 'sizeable'. Interestingly, in her 1975 article 'The Woman Who Isn't Slim Desires High Fashion, Too', Klemesrud uses 'fat' exclusively, unless she is directly quoting someone else.

While language certainly plays a pivotal role in the resignification of the fat female body, it would not be unwarranted to question just how much reclaiming 'fat' can do when the fat body is already imbued with so much meaning, when the fat woman is 'outed' before she can 'out' herself: 'bodies speak, without necessarily talking because they become coded with and as signs … [they] become intextuated, narrativised; simultaneously, social codes, laws, norms, and ideals become incarnated' (Elizabeth Grosz quoted in LeBesco 2004: 6–7). We are taught to understand fat bodies not only as indicators of poor health, but as lazy, having poor hygiene and slow intellect, and lacking willpower (Blaine and McElroy 2002: 351). As fat studies scholar Samantha Murray (2008) maintains, following Foucault, the fat body always already confesses to these 'sins' 'and thus an interior 'truth' is supposedly assigned to the 'fat' subject, for them to then admit and confirm' (75); 'the obligation to confess', writes Foucault, 'is so deeply ingrained in us, that we no longer perceive it as the effect of a power that constrains us'; instead 'confession frees' (quoted in Murray 2008: 75). It is not surprising then, how much of 'The Forgotten Woman' is focused on the fat women themselves 'confessing': what and how much they eat, failed attempts at dieting, and the admission by Mrs. Charles Shipman that she has 'no excuse' for being fat: 'I've always been this big'. This perhaps begs the question: how is this type of (fat-negative) confession different than the seemingly liberatory and fat-positive 'coming out' posed by Sedgwick?

Queer Bodies Queering Fashion

In 1971, *Time Magazine* reported on fat Las Vegas performer Nancy Austin's new line of plus-size clothing 'Pudgy Playmates'. The article, about the surprising success the independent designer was seeing, marvels at the fact that Austin sold 'size 52 hot pants' along with 'gold lame pantsuits, gaucho pants, knickers, and patio dresses' ('Modern Living: Big Business'). While *Time* seems to laud Austin's audacity and her belief that these clothes 'make fat women feel happier', the unnamed author concludes that 'dieting would be a better solution', because the overall 'effect' of happy fat women in hot pants is 'grotesque' (ibid.). This perfectly echoes LeBesco's claim that most people will perceive fat-positive identification as 'grotesque perversion' (2001: 83) and find fat bodies to be 'revolting' (75). However, she argues, 'if we think of *revolting* in terms of overthrowing authority, rebelling, protesting, and rejecting, then corpulence carries a whole new weight as a subversive cultural practice' (ibid.); corpulence, in other words, has the power to *queer* how we think about bodies.

The 'Pudgy Playmates' line of clothing is perhaps a better example of this potential than are Klemesrud's 'forgotten women' – in fact, the line sounds remarkably similar to the contemporary lines put out by independent and queer fat fashion designers.

Finally, we return to Sedgwick's dream and the pink triangle. As a symbol of pride reclaimed by GLBT activists, 'the "pink triangle" that replaces a size number that is necessarily stigmatized is significant, in that it enables Sedgwick to reposition herself positively in relation to pathologising discourses and their histories, to assert some agency in her own *becoming*, to be "extremely cheerful" to become *divine*' (Murray 2008: 97). An analysis of 'The Forgotten Woman' that sees these women as simply reinscribing anti-feminist hierarchies of beauty in their desire to wear high fashion, 'ruffles, ostrich feathers, [and] fox coats' would fail to see the subversive possibilities non-normative bodies bring to the table when they perform in ways that are not socially acceptable. For the thin woman in 1969, refusing to wear makeup and 'letting oneself go' was a wilful subversion of the norm; for the fat woman, *who was already portrayed as such*, demanding access to couture and refusing to wear clothing that camouflaged her corpulence was the very definition of 'queer'. That is to say, while it is certainly true that a desire to be perceived as 'beautiful' stems from the cultural imperative that women *be* beautiful (and thus reproduces, to a certain extent, patriarchal structures), it is possible that because the fat woman always already violates these ideals in her corpulence, the move to appropriate femme fashion and beauty for herself is a necessarily 'queering' endeavour.

The various ways in which fat folks queer fashion and its consumption are even clearer today. Perhaps one of the best examples of this is provided by Charlotte Cooper (2008) in her explanation of The Big Fat Flea (originally Fat Girl Flea) in New York City. The annual fashion event/rummage sale, held at the LGBT Community Centre and benefiting NOLOSE, a fat-positive and queer-centred non-profit, attracts over 500 visitors:

> It builds community and autonomous fat culture across social boundaries, and participants are encouraged to share stories and clothes. It also exposes an archaeology of fat fashion, digging through the stacks of clothes gives a clear picture of what the fashion industry has decided is appropriate garb for fat bodies. Yet at the Flea these rules are subverted, people squeeze into clothes of the "wrong" size, they make things their own, and play dressing-up for the fun of it. This empowers an underclass of people with a pernicious heritage of self-hatred to experiment with kinder and more affirming ways of experiencing our bodies through playing with clothes in a supportive atmosphere. The Flea addresses American consumerism and suggests more environmentally-friendly alternatives. Profits go towards making NOLOSE conferences accessible to people who could not normally attend. (15–16)

In 1969, it was literally *newsworthy* that a fat woman like Mama Cass wore pants, or that Totie Fields allowed herself luxuries only afforded to wealthy thin women, such as fur. Today, while the exact rules have changed (fat women are now allowed to wear pants, but are still encouraged to wear darker 'slimming' colours and avoid horizontal stripes and stretchy fabric), the cultural impetus to follow them remains the same. Fat people who dare to 'squeeze into clothes of the 'wrong' size' and 'make things their own, play[ing] dress-up for the fun of it' continue to subvert oppressive fashion norms and – through alternative consumption events like The Flea and the creation of fashion lines by queer fat designers – potentially queer the industry itself.

When fat women wear clothing that renders them visible in unexpected ways, when they break the 'rules' and 'defy "tasteful" conventions', fashion can be used as a tool to 'stymie fat oppression' (LeBesco 2004: 73). The very fact of a fat woman performing a kind of 'traditional' beauty ('nice' clothes, makeup, and so on.) that she is not supposed to have access to, forces us to rethink culturally-embedded ideas about beauty and even femininity in the first place. Although it is important to be critical of the problematic ways Klemesrud's 'Forgotten Woman' plays into dominant discourses about race, gender, class, sexuality and bodies, it is still possible to understand her as – at least in part – committing truly subversive, even 'revolutionary' acts through her clothing. A far cry from current cultural conceptions of fat consumers, the fa(t)hionista – both in 1969 and today – allows us to analyse fat embodiment, consumption practices, and style in complex and exciting ways.

References

Abelson, E. 1989. *When Ladies Go A-Thieving: Middle-Class Shoplifters in the Victorian Department Store.* New York: Oxford University Press.

Adam, A. 2001. Big girls' blouses: Learning to live with polyester, in *Through the Wardrobe: Women's Relationships With Their Clothes,* edited by A. Guy and E. Green. Oxford: Berg, 39–53.

Blaine, B. and McElroy, J. 2002. Selling stereotypes: Weight loss infomercials, sexism, and weightism. *Sex Roles,* 46, 351–7.

Bordo, S. 1993. *Unbearable Weight.* Berkeley: University of California Press.

Bourdieu, P. 1984. *Distinction: A Social Critique of the Judgment of Taste.* Cambridge: Harvard University Press.

Clark, D. 1991. Commodity lesbianism. *Camera Obscura,* 9(1–2 25–26), 181–201.

Clifford, S. 2010. Plus-size revelation: Bigger women have cash, too. *The New York Times.* [Online, 18 June] Available at: http://www.nytimes.com/2010/06/19/business/19plus.html [accessed 12 October 2011].

Cochrane, K. 2010. Young, fat, and fabulous. *The Guardian*. [Online, 30 January] Available at: http://www.guardian.co.uk/theguardian/2010/jan/30/fat-fashion-blogs [accessed 12 October 2011].

Cooper, C. 2008. What's fat activism? (Working paper WP2008–02). Available at University of Limerick Department of Sociology Working Paper Series website: http://www3.ul.ie/sociology/docstore/workingpapers/wp2008-02.pdf [accessed 3 November 2012].

Farrell, A.E. 2011. *Fat Shame: Stigma and the Fat Body in American Culture*. New York: New York University Press.

Feuer, J. 1999. Averting the male gaze: Visual pleasure and images of fat women, in *Television, History, and American Culture: Feminist Critical Essays*, edited by M. Haralovich and L. Rabinowitz. Durham: Duke University Press, 181–199.

Gerber, L. and Quinn, S. 2008. Blue chip bodies, fat phobia and the cultural economy of body size, in *Bodily Inscriptions: Interdisciplinary Explorations Into Embodiment*, edited by L.D. Kelly. Newcastle: Cambridge Scholars, 1–27.

Hartley, C. 2001. Letting ourselves go: Making room for the fat body in feminist scholarship, in *Bodies Out of Bounds: Fatness and Transgression*, edited by J.E. Braziel and K. LeBesco. Berkeley: University of California Press, 60–73.

Kinzel, L. 2012. Two Whole Cakes. New York: Feminist Press at the City University of New York.

Klemesrud, J. 1969. The forgotten woman in the 'skinny revolution'. *The New York Times*, 1 December, p. 52, accessed 9 June 2011 from ProQuest Historical Newspapers Database (Document ID: 89387415).

Klemesrud, J. 1970. There are a lot of people willing to believe fat is beautiful … *The New York Times*, 18 August, p. 38, accessed 9 June 2011 from ProQuest Historical Newspapers Database (Document ID: 78803213).

Klemesrud, J. 1975. The woman who isn't slim desires high fashion, too. *The New York Times*, 10 April, p. 45, accessed 9 June 2011 from ProQuest Historical Newspapers Database (Document ID: 76552603).

Kuppers, P. 2001. Fatties on stage: Feminist performances, in *Bodies Out of Bounds: Fatness and Transgression*, edited by J.E. Braziel and K. LeBesco. Berkeley: University of California Press, 277–291.

Leach, W.R. 1984. Transformations in a culture of consumption: Women and department stores, 1890–1925. *The Journal of American History*, 71(2), 319–342.

LeBesco, K. 2001. Queering fat bodies/politics, in *Bodies Out of Bounds: Fatness and Transgression*, edited by J.E. Braziel and K. LeBesco. Berkeley: University of California Press, 74–87.

LeBesco, K. 2004. *Revolting Bodies? The Struggle to Redefine Fat Identity*. Amherst, MA: University of Massachusetts Press.

Lupton, D. 1996. *Food, the Body, and the Self*. London: Sage Publications.

Miller, D. 1998. *A Theory of Shopping*. Cambridge: Polity Press.

Modern living: Big business, *Time Magazine*, November 29, 1971. Available at: http://www.time.com/time/magazine/article/0,9171,877469,00.html [accessed 9 June 2001].

Moon, M. and Sedgwick, E. 2001. Divinity: A dossier, a performance piece, a little-understood emotion, in *Bodies Out of Bounds: Fatness and Transgression*, edited by J.E. Braziel and K. LeBesco. Berkeley: University of California Press, 292–328.

Murray, S. 2008. *The 'Fat' Female Body*. New York: Palgrave Macmillan.

Rappaport, E. 2000. *Shopping for Pleasure: Women in the Making of London's West End*. Princeton, NJ: Princeton University Press.

Riggs, C. 1983. Fat women and clothing, an interview with Judy Freespirit, in *Shadow on a Tightrope: Writings by Women on Fat Oppression*, edited by L. Schoenfelder and B. Weiser. Iowa City: Aunt Lute Press, 139–143.

Index

Printed in the United States
by Baker & Taylor Publisher Services